7·8·77

FEELING
FINE

FEELING FINE

A 20-DAY PROGRAM OF PLEASURES FOR A LIFETIME OF HEALTH

by Dr. Art Ulene

Published by J. P. Tarcher, Inc.
Los Angeles

Distributed by St. Martin's Press
New York

ACKNOWLEDGMENTS

Feeling Fine and I owe much to John Fried, whose format ideas contributed greatly to the shaping of this book. Special thanks also go to Victoria Pasternack, Lucy Barajikian, and Brian Williams, whose editorial skills made the finished program even more effective.

Library of Congress Catalog Card No.: 76-29221

Distributor's ISBN: 312-90533-5

Publisher's ISBN: 0-87477-062-9

Designed by Bert Johnson/Graphics Two
Illustrated by Judy Markham
Typography by Graphic Typesetting Service

Manufactured in the United States of America

Published by J. P. Tarcher, Inc.
9110 Sunset Blvd., Los Angeles, Calif. 90069

Published simultaneously in Canada by Macmillan of Canada
70 Bond St., Toronto, Canada M5B IX3

1 2 3 4 5 6 7 8 9 0 / 77 78 79 80

To My Patients,
who shared their secrets for health

To Priscilla, Doug, Val, and Steve,
who shared everything

Contents

DAY 0

Are You Feeling Fine?

- You can't be angry much of the time and feel fine.
- You can't hurt after almost any form of physical exertion and feel fine.
- You can't need pills to calm down or stay awake and feel fine.
- You can't be twenty-five pounds overweight and feel fine.
- You can't feel manipulated by others and feel fine.
- You can't be out of breath after bending to tie your shoes and feel fine.
- You can't get tension headaches almost every afternoon and feel fine.
- You can't be chained to a diet every day of your life and feel fine.
- You can't feel that you are drifting aimlessly through life and feel fine.

This is a book about Feeling Fine.

Feeling Fine means knowing what your feelings are and paying attention to them . . . living in a stressful world without letting it overwhelm you . . . using your body freely and liking the way it feels . . . eating well and enjoying it more. Feeling Fine is growing older and getting better.

Feeling Fine does not mean having the body of Farrah Fawcett or the strength of the Bionic Man. It does not require that you master ancient Oriental meditation techniques or have the habits of a saint. Forget the promises of total fitness. Forget absolute self-control. Forget complete relaxation. Few of us are capable of those states —though we all have the capacity to Feel Fine.

Anyone can do it. But don't expect any book to do it for you. If all it took to make a person healthy in mind, body, and spirit was reading a good book on the subject, we'd be the healthiest people in the world. It takes more than buying a book or even reading a book. If you want to be healthier, if you want to be happier, if you really want to Feel Fine *you have to do it for yourself.*

Feeling Fine involves knowing how to take care of yourself physically, learning to use stress energies constructively, finding ways to express yourself emotionally, and discovering that you can cope with and employ change positively. In order to Feel Fine you have to practice "well-medicine" on yourself. What is well-medicine? It is getting involved with yourself in a program of self-care and self-caring.

You have to take charge of your life. That means accepting the responsibility for keeping yourself healthy and maybe making adjustments in the way you treat your body. It also means making some changes in the way you handle stress and in how you think about yourself. But it doesn't mean you have to stop enjoying food or spend an hour jogging at 6 A.M. every day. Nor does it mean you should shut yourself away from all stressful situations. You don't have to give up all the things that give you pleasure or miss all social contact, but you will need to spend a little time learning where the pleasure in your life really comes from and finding out the price you pay for it.

You can't be a bystander in your own body, sitting idly on the sidelines while your body battles the hazards of your particular style of living. You can't neglect the maintenance of your body and expect it to function well. You can't abuse your body for years and expect a doctor to patch you up in a day. A few prescriptions may get you back on the field of battle, but your body will never be the same. Getting a clean bill of health on the annual physical exam doesn't mean you're healthy. By the time the doctor can find something wrong with you, things may have gone too far.

This book is designed to help you practice well-medicine. It is filled with hundreds of suggestions for activities that will leave you feeling healthier and happier. This is not a book you read. This is a book you DO. It is a book you LIVE. This is not my book, it is yours.

Do it. Live it. And soon you'll be Feeling Fine.

The Feeling Fine Program

• If you cough all the time from smoking, losing twenty pounds won't leave you Feeling Fine.

You cannot mistreat one aspect of your being without causing disharmony in others. Ignore one of your parts and something goes wrong with the rest.

• If everyone at home makes you angry, running three miles a day won't leave you Feeling Fine.

Nothing that takes place in your mind can fail to have some effect on your body. No significant activity in your body will take place without having some effect on your mind. The effects may be small—so small you may not even be aware of them—but they will be there. And when they are bad for one part of your body, they will be bad for all of you.

• If you are not aware of your emotions, learning to meditate won't leave you Feeling Fine.

Enjoying meditation in a tension-provoking world is a great idea, but learning to recognize and deal successfully with the root causes of your stress may even be a better place to start. A sense of inner peace and profound self-knowledge may be hard to obtain, but there are readily available techniques you can use to help you find your way.

Feeling Fine is not a handbook on meditation, although it will teach you how to relax. It's not a diet program, although it will show you how to eat better. It's not an exercise program, although it will show you how to bring your body to vigorous life. It's not a program of emotional therapy, but it will help you get in touch with your feelings.

This is a book for your total being. It deals with your physical side and your emotional side: how to nurture them and make them feel good. We'll also consider the world around you, since your environment cannot help but affect your world within.

Feeling Fine is not the result of a single act. You can't diet yourself, exercise yourself, or even relax yourself into it. It is a sum total of attitudes and behaviors, of physical, emotional, and mental well-being. So, as you read through the twenty-day program don't be surprised when you find a lot of overlap. It's intentional.

The material in this book is divided into four general categories:

• Growing Pleasures   • Eating Pleasures
• Unstressing Pleasures   • Body Pleasures

Why does each of the sections contain the word *pleasures?* Because pleasuring yourself is the most consistent theme of this program. Life should be a pleasure—not a constant state of self-denial. The full enjoyment of life is the best prescription I know for staying healthy. And the health of your total being depends on the health of your individual parts.

Body Pleasures is not just about how your body looks and feels. Limber your body and you'll feel less pain. Feel less pain and you'll sleep with fewer interruptions. Sleep with fewer interruptions and you'll awake more refreshed. Awake more refreshed and you'll anger less easily. Anger less easily . . . . The chain never ends and you feel better and better. Before you know it, you're Feeling Fine.

Growing Pleasures is about a lot more than just recognizing and responding to your feelings and desires. Express your feelings and you'll feel less frustration. Feel less frustration and you'll spend less time angry. Spend less time angry and your body will be more relaxed. Relax your body and your headaches may disappear. Are you beginning to see the connections?

You won't find any miraculous cures in this book, no "great discoveries," no wild claims. You will find the best health ideas and practices I could gather from authorities around the world, some ancient wisdom, some modern discoveries, and a lot of common sense. Some of the most useful advice in the book comes from my patients and other generous people who have shared their experiences with me on television. Their advice is not theoretical, it's based on success in real life. You may have heard some of it before and not done anything about it. This time I hope you will give it a try.

For the next few pages I'll explain briefly what you can expect to find in each of the four general categories I listed. After reading through each description you'll find specific instructions on how to use the twenty-day program that follows. In just a few minutes you'll be ready to start the program.

The Feeling Fine Pleasures

GROWING PLEASURES

If you watch my segment on the "Today" show, you know that I spend a lot of time trying to demonstrate the alternative to growing older. It's growing *better*. Week after week there are men and women on the program who prove the point. These people never stop learning new techniques for *living*. Ask any of them and he or she will tell you, "Life gets better every year."

Why does life get better? Because *they* get better at extracting pleasure from life. They learn how to set personally meaningful goals and how to achieve them. They learn to change loneliness into serenity and feelings into action. They learn to express anger as well as affection, to live with a plan as well as to be spontaneous. They know how to satisfy the many different and conflicting needs of their own personality.

These people prove that learning doesn't stop when you leave school, growing doesn't stop when you finish puberty, and life doesn't end when you leave your youth. They teach us that the best part of life lies ahead, if we are willing to change as life changes. That's what the Growing Pleasures section of this book is all about.

What can you expect to find in Growing Pleasures? Expect to think about who you are and why you act the way you do. And expect to act with a greater sense of freedom as a result. Expect to learn techniques for setting and for achieving goals—and to reach some goals in the process. Expect to find some new ways to solve old problems. Expect to hunt for old treasures and to find new pleasures. Expect to break old habits and to find new freedoms. Expect to think about changing and to change as you do. And expect to Feel Fine.

Here is a list of the Growing Pleasures you'll be discovering:

UNSTRESSING PLEASURES

Your heart pounds, your blood pressure rises, your hormones surge, you can't sleep. These are natural responses to stress, and they won't hurt you unless they happen all the time. Then the pounding becomes palpitations, the rapid pulse becomes a tachycardia, the rise in blood pressure becomes hypertension, sleeping difficulties become insomnia. The natural responses to stress become disease.

You don't necessarily have to feel stressed to be stressed. Stress can become so habitual that you don't even know you're suffering from it. Our bodies learn to accept constantly higher levels of tension until they become pained and sick. Our psyches learn to live with constantly higher levels of stress until they become anxious and depressed.

Often the difference between health and illness is being able to turn off the stress response. It's one of the keys to your becoming a practitioner of well-medicine.

Family physicians say that stress reactions account for almost 80 percent of the problems they see in their offices. Headaches, stomach pain, rashes, coughs, diarrhea, weakness—no body system or organ is immune. Some doctors prescribe pills by the pound—sedatives to put you to sleep, amphetamines to wake you up, tranquilizers to quell your anxiety, and narcotics to kill your pain. Before long the side effects of the treatment are as bad as (or worse than) the original disease.

Test after test is ordered, seeking any cause. Operation after operation is performed, seeking any cure. Still the patient returns. The problems persist. Sadly, many physicians don't even recognize that stress is the root of the trouble.

Is stress unavoidable? Perhaps not. There are times when it seems almost impossible to get out of bed without confronting a stressful situation.

Do we need to get sick over it? Absolutely not. And we don't need to subject ourselves to the dangers of drugs or alcohol to deal with it, either. Popping a Valium is not the way to find health and happiness.

The alternatives are surprisingly simple. Eliminate unnecessary stress. Protect yourself against the physiological changes that come with stress. Cancel those changes when they do occur.

What can you expect to find in the Unstressing Pleasures section? Expect to learn where your stress is coming from and to find out how to recognize when you're under stress by identifying your own "target organs." Expect to learn how to use techniques like autogenics, guided imagery, and meditation to restore your stressed body systems to good health.

Expect to learn the tricks of better sleep and to wake up feeling fresher when you put those tricks to work. Expect to find an "inner adviser" and to get some free advice when you do.

Expect to deal better with stress in your life and to gain the sense that, by taking charge of your stress you can take charge of other aspects of your life. Expect to find yourself Feeling Fine when you do.

Below are the twenty days of Unstressing Pleasures that you will experience:

DAY 1   Your Target Organs
DAY 2   Stress: Finding Your Triggers
DAY 3   Removing the Causes of Stress
DAY 4   Removing Yourself from the Stress
DAY 5   Returning Stress to Its Rightful Owner
DAY 6   Easing Stress with Guided Imagery
DAY 7   A Place of Your Own
DAY 8   Finding a Friend with Guided Imagery
DAY 9   Guided Imagery and Pain Relief
DAY 10 Preparing for Sleep
DAY 11 When You Have Trouble Sleeping
DAY 12 It's All in the Muscles
DAY 13 Rock-a-bye Baby
DAY 14 Patient, Heal Thyself
DAY 15 Autogenics: Breathing

EATING PLEASURES

Fifty million people are overweight. Millions more suffer with atherosclerosis, anemia, and a long list of other diseases related to what they eat and don't eat.

Most of us are overfed and at the same time undernourished. Almost everyone is on a diet; almost no one is happy about it. In one way or another eating is just about everybody's problem.

I like eating so much I once worked my way up to 201 pounds. Trouble is, I didn't feel fine when I got there. I've lost 30 pounds since then, and I didn't do it by dieting. I lost the weight by changing the way I ate.

In 1976 when I began my television series, "Feeling Fine," in Los Angeles, I started with almost everybody's problem—eating.

For twenty days we talked about the joy and benefits of eating well, and we showed people new ways to eat. We focused on a young couple as they began to eat differently. As their eating patterns changed, right in front of our eyes their appearance improved, their energy increased, they felt better about themselves. Eventually, as the program was aired in New York, Chicago, Cleveland, and Washington, millions of viewers wrote in for a brochure that outlined the Feeling Fine Eating Plan. Hundreds of thousands lost weight. Everyone had fun. That fun is what you can expect in the Eating Pleasures section.

Expect an eating program as much for people who are underweight or overweight as for those at their right weight.

Expect to learn more about the foods you eat, the differences between those that harm your body and those that enhance your health. Expect to eat better as you do. Expect to find out why you sometimes eat when you're not hungry and how you can stop it; how you can shop in ways that will automatically make your eating habits more healthful; how you can get satisfaction at the table without putting your fork in your mouth.

We'll show you how to make less food look like more and tell you how more food can actually have fewer calories.

This is not a specialized diet. Instead this program contains literally hundreds of suggestions for eating better and enjoying it more. Our object is not to take the pounds off—although if you are overweight that will happen as you learn new ways to eat. The object is to increase the benefits and pleasures you get when you eat.

While you wend your way through Eating Pleasures you'll find new ways to eat and, as you do, you can also expect to find yourself Feeling Fine.

This is your program of Eating Pleasures:

DAY 1   Growing Better, Not Bigger
DAY 2   Calories: Finding the Thin Ones
DAY 3   The SCS Plan: Substituting
DAY 4   The SCS Plan: Cutting
DAY 5   The SCS Plan: Skipping
DAY 6   Trimming the Fat
DAY 7   Fiber: Slip Me Some Skin
DAY 8   Sugar: Cut Out the Sweet Talk
DAY 9   Liquor: Handle with Care
DAY 10   Vitamins: The ABCs of Good Health
DAY 11   Additives: Not Quite Fresh-off-the-Farm

BODY PLEASURES

You own the world's greatest pleasure machine. It's your body. Maintain it well, and it will take you almost anywhere you want to go. Rest it well at night, and it will make you feel good in the morning. Scratch its back, and it will make you feel great all over. All you have to do is treat it right.

You probably think I'm working my way up to the word *exercise*. Wrong. I said *pleasure*, and that's what I meant. Everyone has tried exercise already, and almost everyone has given up on it. It's not that they haven't tried hard enough. In most cases they've tried too hard. They push themselves until they hurt—so they stop. They drive themselves until they're tired—so they stop. They do the same things over and over until they're bored —so they stop.

Basically, people stop exercising because they're not having fun while they're doing it, and the long-range rewards—a stronger heart, a longer life, a better figure —are just too far away to keep them at it.

We're going to introduce you to a different concept. Don't concentrate on the long-term goals; they'll take care of themselves. Concentrate instead on the pleasure to be found in the process. It's there when you look for it, and the best way to do that is to pay full attention to the experience while you are making it happen. That way you won't get discouraged waiting for a reward; the process itself will be rewarding. You won't get bored, you won't get tired, you won't get hurt. Most important, you won't feel like quitting.

A number of the Body Pleasures experiences bring your senses to life—self-massage, mutual massage, dancing, and bathing. They will help you become more aware of your body and of the many ways it has of Feeling Fine.

As you discover the Body Pleasures, expect to move your joints a little more than you have been doing. Expect them to move a little better as a result. Expect to stretch some muscles you've been neglecting. Expect them to relax a little better as a result. Expect to walk more, breathe deeper, and move with an ease you may not have felt for years. Expect to learn about endurance—you may even make it a goal in your life.

Expect to find a lot of pleasure in your body. You won't be disappointed.

These are the twenty days of Body Pleasures that await you:

DAY 1   Make Life Sense-sational
DAY 2   Self-Massage: Get a Grip on Yourself
DAY 3   Mutual Massage: Sharing the Fun
DAY 4   Take a Deep Breath
DAY 5   Step Right This Way
DAY 6   It's What's Up Back That Counts
DAY 7   Limbering Up to Save Your Neck
DAY 8   Limbering Up to Save Your Shoulders
DAY 9   Limbering Up to Save Your Hips
         and Knees

Throughout this section I've been telling you what to expect. I honestly believe that all the good things I've mentioned are available to anyone who really gets involved in the Feeling Fine Program. I would be less than honest, though, if I didn't say a few words on what *not* to expect.

Don't expect instant anything. Don't expect to master any technique, such as autogenics, assertiveness, stretching, meditation, or dream working, from just two or three days of practicing it.

Feeling Fine is in many ways an introduction to some of the most effective techniques available to anyone who wants to find new ways to enjoy life and get what they want out of it. But the experiences in this book are only a beginning. So I've included a suggested reading list keyed to the four major "pleasures" we'll cover in this book.

Using the Program

Some people buy every new diet book published. They just buy them, they don't read them. They put them on the shelf and hope that somehow *buying* books will make them thinner. My professional opinion is that it never does.

Some people read every new self-awareness book that's published. They just read the books, they never follow the advice. They keep hoping that *reading* the books will do the job. It never does.

Putting *Feeling Fine* on your shelf won't make you feel fine. Just reading *Feeling Fine* won't make you feel fine, either. You're going to have to *do* the program if you want it to do anything for you.

In each of the twenty days you'll find many recommended activities from which to choose. You don't need to do them all to feel fine. But you should try to do *at least* one from each category every day. That's the best way to insure some balance as you work at developing a more healthful way of life.

Some of the activities require almost no effort and may seem unimportant. Do them anyway. Do them first, judge them later. Some may seem too large to tackle. Don't shy away because of that. At least for the next twenty days, make a commitment to try almost anything once.

Even if you tried something similar before and it didn't work, try it again. You're not the person you were when you tried it last, and this time the pieces may fall into place. If they don't, there are lots of other things to do.

If you find an activity that really turns you on (and there should be plenty of them here), don't be afraid to do a lot more of it, even if it uses up a lot of your time.

If you find something that really turns you off, don't do it at all, even if you've got nothing but time.

Different readers will find it easier to get involved with some techniques than with others. For example, I have always found it easy to do guided imagery and much harder to do meditation, but you may find exactly the opposite to be true for you. If you are not getting good results from a technique—if you've given it a good chance to help you feel fine and it just doesn't seem to be doing it—don't decide that the whole area is not for you. Just move forward to the next technique in that area and give it a try.

If you develop just one good technique from Unstressing Pleasures, you will have helped yourself feel better. If you change just some of your eating habits, you will move toward greater health. The same is true for Growing Pleasures and Body Pleasures. Nothing that you learn here will be wasted if you make it part of your life.

Don't limit yourself to the activities listed in the book. Create new ones for yourself. Invent and enjoy. Don't try to squeeze yourself into something that doesn't fit.

Take this program and make it yours.

Doing the Program

The Feeling Fine Program is designed to take twenty days. The benefits should last a lifetime. That's not a bad investment.

In each pleasures section (Growing, Unstressing, Eating, Body) you'll find some facts to acquaint you with the topic we're covering that day and activities to do afterward. The activities are what this book is all about.

When you've finished reading the material for any given day, you're done with the book for the day. But you're not done with the program. Then it's time to do the activities that have been suggested. As much as possible we have chosen activities that can be done as soon as you've finished reading. Others you'll have to make time for in your day.

Many of the activities will require no extra time in your life. Since you've got to take time to eat, it takes no longer to eat well. The same can be said for sleeping, bathing, and even breathing—all topics on which we have some suggestions.

Many of the activities, such as those covered in the sections called "Time Alone," "The 'No' That Says 'Yes'," "Guided Imagery for Problem Solving," "Sleeping On It," and many more, will actually add extra minutes to your day.

If it seems as if you don't have any time, you'll find plenty of tips throughout the book that will show you where you can find it. Ideally, try to set aside a specific time each day when you'll do your reading and try the activities. That's the best way to insure that you give the program enough time to work for you.

What if you have a little extra time and you want to read ahead? Resist the urge. Don't rush. This isn't a competition. If you allow the program to span the full twenty-day period and concentrate on each experience as you do it, the activities are more likely to become a part of your life.

If you really want to do more and you have extra time, go backward. Read something over again. *Do* something over again. Try an activity you skipped or slighted or that didn't seem to work out the way you expected the first time. This is a program for living, which is something you do every day.

What if you miss a day? Or two? Or three? Don't

despair. And don't give up. This isn't the kind of program that you have to do every day or you go back five paces. It took you twenty, thirty, forty, maybe fifty or more years to get where you are and become who you are; a few extra days to make some changes you'd enjoy aren't going to make any difference.

I know how valuable all the things I'm recommending in this book can be. I've tried them out and enjoyed them. I also know that days (and sometimes many days) go by without my having any of the body-pleasuring experiences that I recommend. There are times when I get very stressed and don't deal with it in the ways that I suggest you deal with it. Certainly there are days when my eating habits are not what I know they should be. But that doesn't mean that I shouldn't go back to the desired behaviors as soon as I possibly can. I try to do them more often than not, and more often than not I succeed. Indeed I'm succeeding more often as time goes by.

I know I'm not involved in a discipline like an Olympic athlete, spending all of my emotional and physical energy to perfect certain capabilities. My life—and yours, I'm sure—is too complicated for that kind of dedication. It is not too complicated, however, to incorporate as many of these experiences into my daily living as I can. It is not too complicated for me to be aware of the alternative experiences that this book is suggesting and to practice them whenever I can.

So if you miss a couple of days—or even weeks —just add that to your timetable and pick up the program right where you left off.

Feeling Fine Points

The real reward for doing the *Feeling Fine* program is FEELING FINE. This book emphasizes immediate rewards as well as long-term benefits. The Body Pleasures that we suggest are fun to do when you are doing them, and they also deliver the long-term benefits of greater health. The Unstressing Pleasures should make you feel better almost from the very beginning, and the Growing Pleasures and Eating Pleasures are meant to bring you immediate satisfaction and lifelong benefits.

There's another reward you don't have to wait for, something you can give yourself every day—Feeling Fine points.

Every time you complete one of the recommended activities during the twenty days of the program you earn a point. Every day you'll find new ways to earn points. Any time you repeat an old activity you can earn an extra point. (Some days you'll be tripping all over the points you earn. Other days points may seem a little harder to come by. Slowly but surely your point total will grow.)

To make it easy to keep track of your points there's a "point page" at the end of each day in the program. On that page the point activities for the day are printed in **bold type**; reminders of past point-earning activities are in regular type. (Leaf ahead and you'll see what a point page looks like.)

What good are the points? Are points just a gimmick? Yes and no. Yes because they won't do you any good in themselves. No because they're proof that you're doing things that are good for you—and sometimes it's helpful to see that in black and white.

The points will tell you how well you are balancing your efforts among the various categories of the program. If all your points are stacking up in the Body Pleasures boxes and no points are appearing in any of the other sections, you're not getting as much as you can out of *Feeling Fine*.

Most important, points are a way of reminding yourself about the Feeling Fine program throughout the day, even when the book isn't in your hand. They are a reminder to you of the many ways in which you can help yourself feel fine simply by enjoying some of the activities suggested each day.

Does it really pay to earn the points? You bet. I can't guarantee how you'll feel if you earn all the possible points in the book, but one thing I'll say for sure: it's not possible to earn points without feeling better.

The Ultimate Reward

It won't take you long to realize that the ultimate reward for doing the Feeling Fine Program is Feeling Fine. And you'll want to do the program for its own sake rather than for points or praise. "Getting there," as the slogan says, "is half the fun."

Do it with as much involvement and concentration as you possibly can. Don't worry about the goal of any specific activity. Give up thoughts of winning or losing, of competing with somebody else—or even with yourself. Suspend all judgments. You can even forget the many things I've told you to expect from this book. Put success and failure out of your mind. There's no way to fail this program unless you stop now.

Just do it, enjoy it, and you'll be Feeling Fine. I promise you.

DAY 1

Growing Pleasures

TABOO TABOOS

- Did you ever want to read a book in bed all night, but found yourself turning out the lights at 11:30?
- Did you ever want to see three movies in the same day, but ended up going to only one?
- Have you ever wanted to order white wine with roast beef, but found yourself sipping red?
- Have you ever wanted steak for breakfast, but wound up cooking eggs?
- Did you ever want to use a first name, but heard yourself saying "Doctor" instead?

We all live with such restrictions. Some of them seem so "natural" that we don't even recognize them for what they really are—unnecessary blocks to freedom and spontaneity. These restrictions may have been appropriate when we were children, but too often we have carried them right into adult life without realizing they are no longer applicable to our adult circumstances.

Now is the time to break out of these patterns—the habits and taboos that inhibit us from Feeling Fine.

Remember when you received your first set of crayons and a coloring book? After an hour or so the book was probably filled. That's when you may have set off to "make your mark" in other books that were lying around. When you got caught there was no praise for your colorful work. Instead you got a lecture about the evil of writing in books. You may even have gotten your bottom warmed.

That sanction against writing in books made sense when you were three—or thirteen. It was a necessity with schoolbooks that other students would use. But it doesn't make sense now when you're using books you've bought for yourself. In fact there are lots of times when it's a *good* idea to write in a book. Underline a passage that is particularly meaningful and you'll be able to find it again. Jot down an idea in the margin and you won't forget what you want to remember. There's nothing *wrong* with adding your own creative work to a printed page.

That's why, unless this is a library book, I want you to write your name in it. By writing your name in this book you will accomplish two things. First it will show that this is no longer my book, it's yours. Second you will have taken a small step toward breaking one of those unnecessary taboos that restrict your life and make it less fulfilling than it could be. Don't be bashful: if this is your book, write your name in the space below. (Your mother will probably never know you did it.) Give yourself one Feeling Fine point for writing your name right here:

_____

(Here and there throughout *Feeling Fine* you'll be asked to write something on these pages. If this is a library book, please disregard those instructions and use a separate sheet of paper. Writing in this book has no secret power, but writing something down—which makes it specific and memorable—sometimes does.)

Now for the second activity for the day: become conscious of other taboos that affect your life. Take a moment to think about the things you've wanted to do but never did.

On this page or on a separate piece of paper list the taboos you'd like to break. They might be small things, similar to the ones I've mentioned. Or, better yet, big things—like not talking to strangers even when you'd love to or not doing something you really want to do because women (or men) simply don't do such things.

PERSONAL TABOO LIST

1. _____

2. _____

3. _____

4. _____

5. _____

6. _____

Keep your personal taboos in mind. If this is your book, tear out the page you've listed them on and carry it with you. (And please don't let tearing pages out of books that belong to you be another one of your taboos.) Then, today, tomorrow, or anytime—give yourself a Feeling Fine point for breaking a taboo.

Unstressing Pleasures

YOUR TARGET ORGANS

Got a headache? Your body may be trying to tell you something.

Backache? Sweating? Itching? There's probably a message there for you.

Stomachache? Muscle spasm? Nervous tic? What is your body trying to say?

The answer is simple: *stop the stress*. These symptoms are your body's natural way of telling you there's too much stress in your life. Everyone has a spot in the body—a special "target organ"—that cries out when stress is too great. The stomach reacts with acid; the arteries, with angina; the breathing passages, with asthma. The target of stress can be the bladder, the skin, or the eyes. Literally no body organs or functions are spared. Whatever the location, the process is the same. Stress attacks your target organs and they cry out for help. The symptoms are all different, but the message is the same: *stop the stress*.

Act on the message in time and the symptom goes away. Ignore the signal and you've set the stage for real physical damage. Let the acid run strong enough and you'll soon have an ulcer. Let the sneezing go on long enough and you'll soon have an asthma attack. Let the chest pain come frequently enough and a heart attack won't be far behind.

During the next twenty days I'll be showing you how to deal with stress more effectively—how to avoid it and how to cancel the harmful effects it has on your body. Today, however, we're going to concentrate on the key to the stress problem: recognizing when you've got it. You'll learn how to identify your own target organs and the signals they send you. Once you're tuned in to these signals you'll be able to recognize stress when it starts to take a toll on your body.

To help you identify your target organs I've prepared a list of some stress reactions doctors commonly see in their patients.

At one time or another I've seen every one of

Common Stress Reactions

Headache	Muscle spasms	Diarrhea
Nervous tics	Itching	Frequent urination
Blurry vision	Excessive sweating	Dermatitis
Dizziness	Palpitations	Hyperventilation
Fatigue	Rapid heart rate	Irregular heart rhythm
Cough	Impotence	High blood pressure
Wheezing	Pelvic pain	Delayed menstruation
Backache	Stomachache	Vaginal discharge

these reactions in patients of mine. These complaints are not always related to stress. Most of them could be caused by organic disease—bacteria, viruses, or toxins, for example—as well as by stress. But when they occur again and again, and the tests fail to show any organic cause, it's time to suspect that stress may be the culprit.

If you don't see any symptoms on the list that you'd call your own, don't think you are necessarily stress free. I may simply have left out your stress reaction. For example, I didn't list hair twisting, fist clenching, jaw tightening, nail biting, and other stress responses that people don't usually go to see a physician about. If you have one or two tension-related complaints that weren't on the list, write them down.

What do you do with this information? Start by paying attention to it. Listen to your body signals and hear what they are saying about the way you live. Open up the lines of communication from your body to your mind. Later on in *Feeling Fine* we'll be sending messages the other way. Your mind will be telling your body to do some pretty surprising things—and surprisingly—your body will be doing them.   1967279

Tomorrow we will look at some possible causes of your stress. Until then give yourself a Feeling Fine point for recognizing when your body tells you it's there.

Eating
Pleasures

GROWING BETTER, NOT BIGGER

If you were watching the "Today Show" in the fall of 1976 you saw it for yourself. Carol and Norb Orens, a couple who are typical of millions of adult Americans, began an eating program which allowed them to get rid of extra pounds and yet eat with more pleasure than they had ever done before.

Norb started the program weighing 220 and lost thirty-seven pounds in fourteen weeks. Carol wouldn't reveal what she weighed at the start but said she wanted to lose fifteen pounds. After four months she was down twelve.

The Orenses didn't lose the pounds by dieting. They didn't lose the pounds by going to a fat farm. They didn't give up their favorite foods. They didn't feel deprived. They didn't have to take drastic measures. They didn't risk their health. They lost the weight by incorporating into their daily lives the same information you are going to receive during the twenty days of Eating Pleasures.

This is *not* a diet program. Anyone who goes on a diet must some day go off it. Planned-meal programs are impractical because active human beings can't follow them. Diets of that kind would be effective only if people could be strapped into hospital beds and the food doled out. Even then, 95 percent of those who lost weight would gain it all back as soon as they got out of the hospital. This is true also of weight-watching resorts, where you have the added pain of paying up to $250 for every pound you lose. And, in many cases, the miracle quick-weight-loss diets you find in books are more dangerous than the fat itself. If they really worked we would long ago have become a trim nation.

Right now some of you are saying to yourselves, "This section doesn't apply to me—I'm not overweight." Or you might be in another group, saying, "I'm overweight, but in my case metabolism is the culprit." This program is still for you. Weight loss will take place only if you need it. But weight loss is only one of the benefits to be derived from this eating program. It will enhance your enjoyment of the whole dining process and, at the same time, help you to eat in a healthier manner—equally important aspects of feeling fine.

Besides, no matter what category you're in— underweight, right weight, or overweight—if you're over 25 you will inevitably gain weight in the coming years unless you do something about the amount of food you take in.

After you reach about 25 your body needs less energy because the body's metabolism—its energy-burning machinery—slows down bit by bit. How much? About ten calories every day per year. This is the equivalent of 3,650 calories a year, which equals one pound of body weight. So to maintain a reasonable weight every year past 25 you are going to have to decrease your food intake by ten calories every day—every year.

At age 26 you would need to drop ten calories from what you ate each day when you were 25. At age 27 the body's need for calories drops another ten calories a day. Now you need a total of twenty fewer calories a day than you did two years earlier. By age 35 your body's energy needs will have dropped a hundred calories a day from your twenty-fifth year. That's some 36,500 calories a year. (This process doesn't start at *exactly* age 25 for everyone. For some people it starts at 30, even 35. But sooner or later it starts—for all of us.)

If you failed to begin cutting back, it would

mean that by age 35 you would be many pounds heavier than you were at 25. Keep this up, and the ballooning-out will progress with every advancing year.

But the average person doesn't automatically drop those ten extra calories each year. Most of us continue to eat as though we were still youngsters. That's why more and more of us become overweight as we grow older.

To sum up: if you want to keep your weight at a reasonable level, you have to begin changing your caloric intake. If you are under 25 and not already overweight, you don't have to worry about this yet. If you are over 25, you have to make your decision now.

Some of you may be thinking, "It's already too late."

Wrong—it's never too late, even if all you do is hold your own. If you wish, you can use the tricks the Orenses learned to lose weight. The same techniques will also help you maintain your present weight. Let's look at them.

There are only two ways to solve the problem of the ten calories per day. One is to increase your physical activity. That's a great way to do it. So good, in fact, that we recommend it for everyone (the Body Pleasures section of the book is devoted to it). But we'd like you to try the other way, too—by increasing your mental activity. During the next three days of this program you'll start *thinking* more about three words that will make it easy for you—substituting, cutting, skipping—what we call the SCS Plan.

• *Substituting* means that you change an old food for a new one, one that is more nutritious and less fattening than the food you have been eating.

• *Cutting* means that you decrease the size of the portions you eat.

• *Skipping* means that you skip those foods that add calories without offering much nutritional value.

Sounds simple, doesn't it? Well, it's even more simple than it sounds, because you don't have to do it with everything you eat. I lost eighteen pounds by concentrating all my substituting, cutting, and skipping on a few "target" foods.

In 1974 I skipped all ice cream and cookies (*almost* all—nobody's perfect). I lost eight pounds.

In 1975 I began to cut the amount of cream and sugar I added to my coffee. Five more pounds disappeared.

In 1976 I learned to substitute chicken and fish for beef. Another five pounds gone.

No suffering. No diet. No change in my physical activity. But eighteen pounds melted away.

You can do it, too. All you have to do is select your own "target" foods. During the next three weeks we'll go after them by substituting, cutting, and skipping.

Today's activity is to pick those "target" foods. Set your sights on foods that do the least *for* you and the most *to* you. Pick foods that you really know you can survive without, or that you could do with less of. Here are some examples to help you get started:

Sugar	Liquor and beer
Cookies	Soft drinks
Cake	Jelly and jam
Doughnuts	Potato chips
Pastries	Crackers
Ice cream	Pretzels
Candy	Corn chips
Butter	Sour cream
Meat	Mayonnaise
Sauces	Peanut butter

Now make your own list. Pick one or two "target" foods to concentrate on for each week of the program.

Week		"Target" Foods
One	1.	_____
	2.	_____
Two	1.	_____
	2.	_____
Three	1.	_____
	2.	_____

Give yourself a Feeling Fine point for writing them down—and avoiding them as often as possible.

Body Pleasures

MAKE LIFE SENSE-SATIONAL

When is the last time you really paid attention to your five senses?

When is the last time you concentrated on using them for pleasure?

How often do you touch—without feeling? Eat—without tasting? Breathe—without smelling?

How often do you look—without seeing? Listen —without hearing?

Most of the time your senses are asleep. You turn them off so they won't distract you from the tasks you are doing.

Today your activity will be to turn those senses back on so you can discover the sensual pleasures that await you. As the first step in awakening your body to the pleasures that lie within, we will wake up your senses to the pleasures in the world around you.

Here are some ideas on how to begin. Don't be afraid to make up your own.

AWAKEN AND PLEASURE YOUR TASTE

1. Cut cubes out of four different kinds of cheese. Mix them up and close your eyes. Can you name the cheeses by taste, without looking?
2. Drink a glass of water. Keep sipping until you can describe how it tastes.
3. Place a drop of honey or lemon on the tip of your tongue. Taste it. Think about what words you would use to describe it.
4. Put five drops of your favorite liquor on your tongue. Taste it. Does it really taste good?
5. Cut a good piece of fruit or a fresh vegetable into slices. How does it taste when you eat it that way?

AWAKEN AND PLEASURE YOUR EARS

1. Close your eyes and count how many different sounds you can hear in three minutes.
2. Turn on a good music station or play your favorite vocalist on a record. This time, try to hear the background music only, not the vocalist. Close your eyes. Can you hear better?
3. Listen to a TV program with the picture covered up or your eyes closed. Can you follow the story? Does the music set the mood?
4. Put a clock under your pillow and listen to the ticking. Concentrate harder. Does it get louder?
5. Listen to instrumental music. Can you pick out the violins or the saxophones?
6. Run the bath and listen to the water as it fills the tub.

AWAKEN AND PLEASURE YOUR EYES

1. Close your eyes. What do you see on the inside of your eyelids? Press your lids ever so gently. Does the scene change?

2. Open your eyes wide. Stare straight ahead. How far can you see to each side? How far to the sides do you usually see?

3. Find an oil painting. Look for the detail. Can you see the brush strokes?

4. Look at a familiar surface—a door, a leaf, the back of your hand. Look closely. How many things are there that you never "noticed"?

AWAKEN AND PLEASURE YOUR NOSE

1. Open your spice cabinet and take out a half dozen jars. Close your eyes. Smell each one separately. See how long it takes you to distinguish among them without looking at the labels.

2. Savor some food aromas. Try a box of crackers, a bag of fruit, a piece of cheese, a fresh can of coffee. Hold them close to your nose. Close your eyes. Are you smelling something for the first time?

3. Put some after-shave lotion, deodorant, or cologne on the back of your wrist. Smell it.

AWAKEN AND PLEASURE
YOUR WHOLE BODY

1. Get someone you like to scratch your back.

2. Stand in a strong wind and feel the wind blow through your hair. Close your eyes and turn slowly in a circle. From which angle do you enjoy the feeling of the wind the most?

3. Gently massage your temples for a few minutes. Which spot provides the most relaxation?

4. Get a feather and find the most sensitive part of your body. Did you ever think it would be there?

5. Set your hair dryer on "cool" or "warm" (not "hot") and direct the stream of air all over your naked body. Better yet, let someone else hold the dryer. Where does it feel best?

These are but a tiny fraction of the opportunities waiting to stroke your senses. Try some. Try them all. Find your own.

Next time you go for a walk, *really listen* to the sounds in the street. Look carefully at things about you. Feel your feet as they touch the sidewalk. Smell the air. Feel the wind.

What's the point of all this sensing? Nothing cosmic. You won't reach a new level of consciousness through your nose. You may not even enjoy some of the sensations. However, if you concentrate on your senses—even for brief periods of time—you'll discover many pleasant sensations are awaiting you.

Wake up your senses. And give yourself a Feeling Fine point every time you do.

FEELING FINE POINTS
(Choose one or more from each category.)

GROWING PLEASURES

☐ **Breaking a taboo**

UNSTRESSING PLEASURES

☐ **Locating a target organ**

EATING PLEASURES

☐ **Picking your target foods**

BODY PLEASURES

☐ **Awakening your senses**

DAY 2

Growing Pleasures

THE "NO" THAT SAYS "YES"

Not long ago my oldest son, Doug, made a comment that changed my life.

"I never see you," he complained, one evening when I came home late. I made an excuse about all the things I had to do, and he went off to bed, seemingly satisfied. But his simple remark still troubled me.

Later that evening a woman called and asked me to speak at a meeting of her charitable organization, and my thoughts returned immediately to Doug and his complaint. Another night away from home. Another night he wouldn't see me. But I couldn't say no, could I? I had to accept. But then Doug's remark made the decision for me.

"I'm sorry," I said. "I can't do it." I was saying yes, not to the lady but to Doug and myself. Without a moment's hesitation she asked, "Can you suggest someone else?" I gave her a few names and realized—painfully, for a moment—I wouldn't be missed.

The night my speech was to have been delivered I was at home, enjoying myself with my family. Saying no to the lady was indeed saying yes to myself.

It's hard to say no to others, to limit the demands they make on us, but it's something we all should learn to do. You don't have to take a course in assertiveness training to start to learn how. That's what this day is all about.

Oddly, the first thing you have to do is recognize that there are times when you *can't* say no. We all have obligations, duties, and responsibilities. Spouses, children, other relatives, bosses, fellow workers, and neighbors often make reasonable requests that we must accept. It's part of having meaningful, responsible relationships.

However, not every request from these sources and from others falls into that category. Some benefit only the person doing the asking. Meeting those demands may make the other person happy, but it won't leave you feeling fine.

Why, then, when we are confronted by an unreasonable request, do we still find it difficult to say no? Partly because "no" is a word we were taught not to use. When we were very young rebellion earned us a parental warning or a slap. So, many of us stopped saying no. Soon some of us became unable to say it. And this inability to say no became part of the way we live.

Of course there are other reasons why we say yes instead of no. We all want to be liked, to be popular. A new acquaintance asks you out on a night you'd rather stay home. But you say yes because you are afraid you won't be asked again. You want to be liked and you don't want to offend anyone.

Sometimes it's guilt that motivates us. You go because you don't want to make the other person feel bad. *You* end up feeling bad instead.

Whatever the reason, if you often find yourself saying yes to things you really don't want to do, you're adding a lot of stress to your life. Giving in to those demands will make you feel as if your life is controlled by others rather than by you. Those "yeses" create stress; they will make you sick—literally.

So, you've got to start thinking of saying no to someone else as saying yes to yourself. It frees your time to pursue activities you really want to do, things you may now be denying yourself. It makes you feel good. And you don't have to make others feel bad to do it. You can say no without being rude, without losing friends. Today I'll try to show you how.

Before we start let's identify three recent demands that you've said yes to, but that you wish you had turned down. Try to think of the sorts of demands that are apt to be made on you again and again.

Do you have a friend who tries to take up all of your free time, when you'd rather spend part of it reading or with someone else?

Are you bothered by co-workers who always ask you to do their work?

Are you aggravated by a neighbor who always asks you to drive the car pool?

Think about it now. When should you have said no? Take out a piece of paper or write it down here. I should have said no when:

1. _____ asked me to _____.
2. _____ asked me to _____.
3. _____ asked me to _____.

How are you going to say no the next time you want to? Chances are it won't be easy, but there are some techniques that should help.

1. *Prepare yourself.* Practice your response before the occasion arises. Consider a couple of different ways to say no to an unreasonable request. You can just say no—flat out. Or you can suggest an alternative. Whatever your choice, prepare your answer. Say it to yourself just as if you were saying it to the person making the request. Use their name. Say it out loud. Say it over and over, until you become comfortable hearing it. When the time comes, the moment will be much easier to face.

2. *Anticipate the response.* People who are used to asking favors or making demands aren't going to let you off the hook without a struggle. They'll argue. They'll insist. You must be prepared to reply. Practice your response until you're sure you won't back down. Sometimes it helps to practice it with a sympathetic friend.

3. *Be ready to try again.* Learning to say no may take a while. If your first effort still ends up with your doing what you didn't want to do, go back to step 1 and prepare yourself again. You're sure to have another chance to practice saying no.

Learn how to say yes to yourself by saying no to others and take a Feeling Fine point every time you do.

Unstressing Pleasures

STRESS: FINDING YOUR TRIGGERS

If you're like the average person you probably checked off more than one body signal on yesterday's stress list. Chances are you have more than one target organ, too. Recognizing those signals and organs will help you to know when stress is affecting you. But just knowing you've got stress isn't enough—you've got to do something about it. That means you have to know where your stress is coming from.

Your target organs don't give you a clue to where your stress comes from. They only tell you where it's ending up. To learn the source you're going to have to use another organ—your brain. When you do you'll be surprised at some of the events that can trigger stress reactions in you. Take a look at this list of examples:

You lose your job.

There's a death in the family.

Your child is doing poorly in school.

Your husband's new job takes him out of town.

You didn't get invited to a friend's party.

The place where you work is noisy.

The dog next door barks all the time.

You put on six pounds.

Your mother complains you never call her.

A woman gets ahead of you at the department store cash register.

They're jack-hammering in the street outside your home.

You spot a parking space but another driver beats you to it.

The movie you want to see has a line two blocks long.

The restaurant you're in is crowded and the service is slow.

You get a traffic ticket.

You're late for your doctor's appointment.

You get an appointment reminder from your dentist.

The price of gas (or coffee) goes up—again.

You break a shoelace in the rush to leave for work.

You spill wine on your new skirt.

Your check bounces.

Your car needs a complete overhaul.

The lawn needs mowing.

The two eggs on your plate remind you about cholesterol.

The Teamsters go on strike.

There's an earthquake in Turkey.

Just reading that list of events can raise your tension level. *Living* the list, as we all do every day, causes even greater stress. Now read this list:

> You get a promotion.
> Your new car arrives.
> The person you're going with finally agrees it's time to get married.
> Your pregnancy test is positive (negative).
> You plan your vacation trip.
> Your boss praises you on the way you handle clients.
> A new friend invites you to a party.
> Your brother wants to visit you for a week.
> Your friend repays that loan.
> You sign up for golf instruction.
> Your dog has puppies.
> Your daughter is going out on her first date.
> Your favorite ball team wins.
> Your wife starts taking tennis lessons.

Even this "good news" list can cause stress. Can you live up to the requirements of your new job? Will you know anybody at the party? Will someone dent your new car? What about the monthly payments for it? What are you going to do with all those puppies?

No doubt there are some triggers of stress in your life which I haven't mentioned. It's not possible to include them all. But at least the list demonstrates how varied the causes of stress can be. Today, as the next step in reducing the effects of stress on your body, you should make your own stress list. To give you an example, here is a list of the things which are stressing me now:

> My malpractice insurance premium is $13,000 this year (for part-time coverage).
> The tax bill on my home increased 47 percent this year.

No matter how much I plead, my kids continue
   to throw footballs around inside the house.
I never get as much sleep as I'd like.
My neighbor's dog squeezes through the fence
   and poops in my yard.
The fan belt to my power steering keeps slip-
   ping, even though I've had the car in the
   shop several times.
I go to bed in fear that I won't get my wake-up
   call.
My tennis game isn't improving.

Some of the things on my list may not sound
very stressful to you. The fact of the matter is, they are
stressful to *me*. That's why they're on my list. And now
that they're on the list it's a lot easier to do something
about them.

But don't spend time stressing yourself over my
list. Make a list of your own. Don't leave any stress you
can think of off the list. Don't focus only on the typical
stresses like money, work, and family problems. Remember to think about responsibilities to friends, what to
do with your leisure, even the condition of your lawn.

For the next twenty-four hours carry the list
wherever you go and add to it as you recognize other
sources of stress that you forgot to write down. Save the
list. We'll be using it during the next few days as we
work on techniques to help you deal more effectively
with the stress in your life.

Give yourself another Feeling Fine point for
finding your stress triggers.

Eating
Pleasures

CALORIES: FINDING
THE THIN ONES

All you have to do to win another Feeling Fine point is answer the following question: Which of these foods has the most calories?

3 ounces of Wheaties
10 ounces of cottage cheese
4 ounces of hamburger
13 ounces of filet of sole
2 cupcakes without icing
3 tablespoons of butter

Which one did you pick? Believe it or not they're all the same—each one contains 300 calories. This test was not intended to trick you, but to show you how confusing calorie counting can be and how important it is to have at least a little knowledge about calories. We don't want to make the same mistake as the hostess who considerately made a low-calorie salad—and then garnished it with canned onion rings. Nine hundred calories' worth of onion rings!

When we eat we all do some funny things. A friend of mine once devoured a sixteen-ounce steak (1,600 calories) in the belief that meat was "good" for him, calorie-wise. At the same meal he turned down a fifty-calorie slice of bread because, as he put it, "That stuff is loaded with calories."

Calories are not all bad. Calories are a measure of energy, and your body needs energy to keep you going. The problem begins when you take in more calories than your body burns. The trouble is that—despite all the calorie counters that have been sold—many people still don't have any idea how many calories they are taking in.

How many calories do you need? It depends on your age, metabolism, the kind of work you do, and other factors. But, roughly speaking, if you are a reasonably active adult and not overweight you need about fifteen calories a day for each pound of body weight (but never fewer than 1,200 calories a day—no matter how little you weigh).

How can you make good judgments about the amount of calories in food? It helps to visualize calories as coming in two kinds of packages: concentrated and diluted. Once you know the difference, it will make a big difference in your eating choices.

Concentrated calories are those that come in big amounts in small portions of food, usually foods high in animal or vegetable oils and fats: meats, nuts, cream, oil, mayonnaise, butter, margarine, ice cream, cake, cookies, and beans, for example. If you eat enough of these food to fill your stomach, you will have eaten more calories than you can possibly burn. The body will use up what it needs and store the rest—as fat. For every extra 3,500 calories unused and stored your body will add one pound of weight.

Diluted calories are those that come in small amounts in large portions of food, usually foods whose bulk consists of water and fiber. Fruits and vegetables are the best example: lettuce, spinach, carrots, cucumbers, onions, celery, cabbage, watermelon, apples, pears, cantaloupe, honeydew melon, grapefruit. Some soups, like bouillon, are great. Fish isn't bad either.

It doesn't take a lot of cabbage or melon to make you feel full. When you eat a portion you satisfy your hunger and some of your body's needs without overwhelming yourself with more calories than you need.

So if you want to cut down the calories you take

in, one good way is to eat more diluted-calorie foods and fewer concentrated ones.

The little test at the beginning of this section gave you the general idea. The list that follows is another comparison of some common foods and their approximate caloric value.

Meat, Fowl, Fish	*Calories*
Crab, ½ cup, steamed	58
Clams, 4 medium, raw	65
Bacon, 2 strips	92
Beef stew, 1 cup	218
Whitefish, baked or broiled, 8 ounces	250
Turkey or Chicken (without skin), 8 ounces	250
Shrimp, fried, 3½ ounces	285
Salmon, 1 cup, canned	286
Tuna, 1 cup, canned	334
Flank steak, braised, 6 ounces	334
Veal loin chop, 6 ounces	400
Lamb, roast leg, 6 ounces	475
Pork roast, 6 ounces	616
Beef steak, 8 ounces	800

Vegetables	*Calories*
Lettuce, ½ cup	4
Raw mushrooms, ½ cup	10
Cauliflower, ½ cup	15
Green beans, ½ cup	17
Asparagus, 6 spears	20
Carrots, boiled, ½ cup	24
Tomato, 1 regular	33
Peas, ½ cup	60
Corn, 1 ear	70

Potato, 1 baked	90
Broccoli, 2 stalks	94
Lima beans, ½ cup	95
Artichoke, 1 boiled	125

Soups (1 cup)	*Calories*
Consommé	30
Chicken	63
Clam chowder	77
Tomato	79
Cream of chicken	108
Pea	132
Lentil	166
Cream of mushroom	215

Breads and Crackers	*Calories*
Saltines, 2	22
RyKrisp, 1 triple cracker	26
Wheat bread, 1 slice	55-85
Rye, 1 slice	70
Corn bread, 1 square	110
Hard roll, 1	130
English muffin, 1	145
Corn chips, 1 ounce	159

Cereals (1¼ cups)	*Calories*
Corn flakes	110
Cream of wheat	165
All bran	170

Spreads, Dressings (1 tablespoon)	*Calories*
Low-cal salad dressing	20
Grape jelly	50
Salad dressing, regular	50-75
Honey	60

Margarine, whipped	85
Butter	100
Margarine, regular	100
Mayonnaise	100
Peanut butter	100

Desserts	*Calories*
Apricot, 1 fresh	18
Watermelon, ½ cup	21
Strawberries, ½ cup fresh	26
Peach, 1 fresh	40
Cherries, ½ cup fresh	41
Cantaloupe, 1 small	68
Apple, 1 fresh	77
Pineapple, canned, 1 slice	95
Banana	114
Tapioca cream, ½ cup	130
Chocolate ice cream, ¼ pint	136
Eclair	271
Apple dumpling	276
Plain cake with icing, 1 piece	400
French apple pie	447
Sundae	850

It's impractical to try to remember the difference between one food at eighty calories and another at eighty-seven. Acquaint yourself with foods as groups (as in the list above) rather than with individual foods. Then make a list of your favorite foods and spend half an hour with any calorie-counting guide, determining which of them are high calorie, medium calorie, and low calorie. This method will make it much easier to keep track of your calories without actually counting them.

Don't be a calorie fanatic. You don't have to worry with every bite how many calories you are taking in. You don't have to give up *all* high-calorie foods—but

you do have to learn to eat them in smaller portions or
less frequently. Don't be afraid of calories. *Do* be aware of
them.

You've already done your Feeling Fine point-
getting exercise for the day. Your task now is to put this
knowledge to work in your life.

Body Pleasures

SELF-MASSAGE: GETTING A GRIP ON YOURSELF

Question: Which of the following words should always
come to mind when you hear the word "massage"?
a. Parlor
b. Partner
c. Pain
Answer: None of the above. Massage does not need to be
done in a parlor, it does not require a partner, and
should *never* be painful.
Question: Where do you get a massage that isn't painful,
if not from a partner or in a parlor?
Answer: Give it to yourself! As you do so, think of the
word "pleasure," because that's what touching yourself can be—if you do it right.

Today we're going to show you how to do it
right. You'll learn how nice your sense of touch can be
when you use it on yourself. It's called "self-massage." It
feels especially good because you get to feel everything
twice, not just through the part that's being pressed, but
through the part that's doing the pressing as well. Before

you start, here are some tips to make self-massage even more enjoyable.

1. Touch yourself in different ways: push, press, roll, squeeze (but never too hard). Try your fingertips, your palms, the heels of your hands, the heels of your feet. Thump it, bump it, shake it (but don't break it). Try everything—even a vibrator if you've got one.

2. Touch yourself in different places. Don't be afraid to touch anything. As long as it feels good, it's okay to touch. Always be gentle, never make pain.

3. Give yourself some time. This is one thing you don't want to hurry. Shut the door, take the phone off the hook, and get acquainted with yourself.

4. Uncover the part you plan to rub. You want to feel *yourself*, not the fabric in a shirt or skirt. If you want to, take off *all* your clothes. Let the fresh air touch what your fingers miss.

5. Use some body lotion, oil, or powder to smooth the movement of your hands. Less friction means more sensation and *that* means more pleasure.

6. Massage doesn't feel good if it's done incorrectly. Here are a few words of caution.

a. Don't massage any lumps, moles, warts, swellings, or varicose veins.

b. Don't massage an area where you have an injury to a joint or where there is any inflammation or abnormal coloration of the skin.

Are you ready for pleasure? Here's what you do.

KNEE MASSAGE

1. Cup your right hand over your left kneecap and, pressing firmly, move your hand in a circular motion over the knee for 30 seconds.

2. To create pressure, press your left hand over your right one. Try to feel every structure around the

kneecap as you move your hands. Concentrate not only on how your knee feels, but on your hands, too.

3. Repeat the process with your left hand on your right kneecap.

LOWER-LEG RUB

1. Sit on the floor and bring your left knee up so that the sole of your left foot is flat on the floor.

2. Place both hands just under the calf muscle, with your fingertips meeting over your shinbone.

3. Massage your calf muscle on both sides by kneading it between the heels of your hands.

4. Move both hands up to the back of your knee and then down toward your ankle again as you continue to knead.

5. Move your hands so that your thumbs meet over your shinbone and your fingertips are over your calves. This time, let your fingers do the massaging.

6. Repeat the process on your right leg.

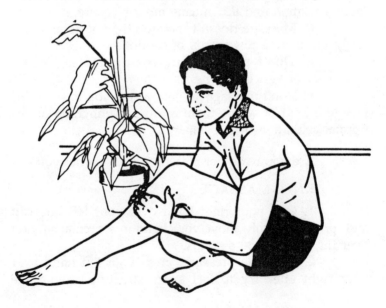

UPPER-LEG RUB

1. Sit in a chair and place the fingers of both hands on the top of your left thigh with your fingers pointing in opposite directions.

2. Slowly move your hands down your leg toward the knee, kneading the flesh on the top of your leg as you go.

3. Move your fingers back along your leg to the top of your thigh. Do this 3 or 4 times.

4. Repeat with your right thigh.

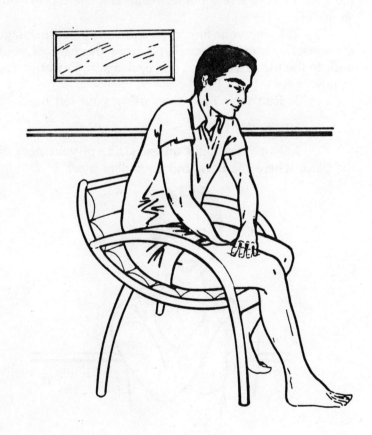

5. Then, moving back to the left thigh, give the outside, inside, and underside of the thigh a massage by repeating this motion. Change the position of your fingers so they can knead the flesh in those areas. Think about how it feels. Do this 3 or 4 times.

6. Repeat with your right thigh.

SHOULDER RUB

1. Place your right palm on your left collarbone so that your fingertips are resting on the muscles between the back of your left shoulder blade and the top of your shoulder.

2. Using your fingertips and your palm, massage the muscles, moving your hand from the base of your neck to the top of your arm and back again. Pay attention to how it feels.

3 Rub your right side, using your left hand.

NECK RUB

1. Place one hand on each side of your neck at the place where the neck and shoulders meet.

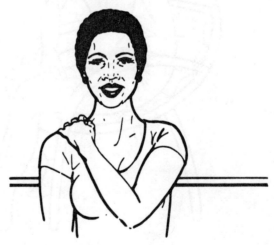

2. Using a circular movement with the fingertips, gently rub the neck for 30 seconds, beginning at the shoulders and moving up to the base of your skull. The massage should cover the back and the sides of the neck.

A nice way to end any self-massage is to shake out your body: stand up and shake your arms, letting them hang loose; next, shake one leg and then the other to get an overall feeling of the release from body tension.

This is just a sampling of some of the self-massage exercises you can do. There is no reason why you can't make up your own, giving other parts of your body the pleasure of your touch.

At the same time, give yourself a Feeling Fine point for taking a few minutes to feel wonderful.

FEELING FINE POINTS
(Choose one or more from each category.)

GROWING PLEASURES
☐ **Saying no to someone, saying yes to yourself**
☐ Breaking a taboo

UNSTRESSING PLEASURES
☐ **Finding the causes of your stress**
☐ Paying attention to your target organs

EATING PLEASURES
☐ **Finding thin calories**
☐ Staying away from your target foods

BODY PLEASURES
☐ **Massaging yourself**
☐ Awakening your senses

DAY 3

Growing Pleasures

REACHING OUT WITH APPRECIATION

I once complimented a friend on giving an exceptionally informative and entertaining talk.

"Do you really think it was good?" he asked.

"Come on," I said. "You know what a good speaker you are."

"I guess so," he replied, "but I still like to be told."

Don't we all.

Most of us rarely hesitate to criticize, even though criticism leaves everyone feeling uncomfortable, and we rarely go out of our way to say something nice, even though that leaves everyone feeling fine. The truth is, reaching out with appreciation is fun—and not just for the person on the receiving end.

I never used to go out of my way to pay compliments. After all, people were supposed to do things well, weren't they? The things I really paid attention to were the things that went wrong. The trouble with that approach was that, by taking the nice things of life for granted, I forgot to respond to them at all.

It took a comment from a valued friend to make

me aware of my problem. He told me how discouraged some of my staff members were because they were putting out their best for me, but my attitude didn't seem to show that I cared or even noticed. My friend, too, wondered whether I cared.

"Of course I care," I answered.

"Then the solution is simple," he replied. "All you have to do is let them know."

I'm trying to change. I'm trying to let others know I appreciate them. (I say "trying" because I don't always succeed.) Sometimes I forget. Sometimes I'm just too busy to notice. Sometimes I'm afraid the other person will misunderstand my motives, so I don't say anything. But I'm trying.

In the past when I received excellent service at a restaurant, I always increased my tip. I still do. But now, in addition, I leave a few kind words, too. "Thanks for making my meal so pleasant."

In the past when a researcher came up with a good topic for our TV segments, I rarely commented on it. That's what researchers are paid to do. Now I try to say, "Thanks. That was a great idea."

In the past when my kids finished practicing their music, I always asked why they didn't practice more. Now I try to tell them how good they sounded. I call this approach "reaching out with appreciation."

A funny thing is happening as I do it. I'm noticing more nice things in my life. Things that go wrong seem less important when compared to all the things that go right. People are more fun to be around. Or—maybe *I'm* more fun to be around.

Reaching out with appreciation isn't hard to do. Here are some more examples of how it works. If these situations don't apply to your life, find your own reasons for doing it. In any case, try to reach out with appreciation today.

• Tell your kids how (smart, funny, enthusiastic, enjoyable, artistic, talented, friendly, kind) they are.

• Tell your wife how (kind, thoughtful, intelligent, sexy, cute, sensitive) she is.

• Tell your husband how (genuine, bright, handsome, sexy, sensitive, clever) he is.

• Tell your co-workers how (productive, helpful, important, creative, responsible) they are.

• Tell your friends how (understanding, supportive, perceptive, fun to be with, interesting) they are.

Look for and pay attention to the nice things about people. Let them know you care. Tell them that you do. Reach out with appreciation and give yourself a little appreciation with a Feeling Fine point.

Unstressing Pleasures

REMOVING THE CAUSES OF STRESS

Two days ago you identified your target organs and the signals they send you. Yesterday you spent time thinking about where your stress is coming from. Today it's time to start doing something about it.

You really have only three choices:

1. You can remove the cause of your stress from the environment.
2. You can remove *yourself* from the stressful environment.
3. You can meet the stress head-on, then try to cancel its harmful effects on your body by using relaxation techniques.

What's the best answer? A combination of all three. During the next seventeen days I'll show you how to use all the techniques, but for the next two days we'll concentrate on how to deal with a stressful environment. Before we start, here are some general principles you can apply whenever you are face-to-face with stress.

Break it up. If the cause of your stress seems too big to tackle, break it up into manageable parts. If your home needed improvement, you wouldn't try to paint all the rooms simultaneously. You'd do them one at a time. If you fell behind on your bills, you wouldn't try to pay them off all at once. You'd set up some kind of install-ment plan. Use the same procedure with the things that are making you tense. Break up your big stress-producing problems into smaller and less tension-provoking ones.

Don't overreact. If someone at work irritates you, a quiet conversation with that person is less stressful than quitting your job. If someone backs into your car, getting it fixed is less stressful than getting into a fight. When you react to stress with drastic measures, your reaction may often cause you more stress than the original prob-lem.

Recognize what can be changed; accept what cannot. Wishing things were different won't make them different and won't make you any more comfortable about the way things are. When nothing can alter an unpleasant or stressful situation, you will find there is a certain peace in acceptance. And much less stress.

Now let's take a look at the best way to cut the stress in your environment. How to do it? Remove it physically.

Does noise bother you? Shut it out, tone it down. Roll up your car windows while you're driving and listen to some quiet music rather than the news—if the news, too, is making you tense. Does the sound of your telephone bell make you jump? Tape the hammer on the bell or put a pad under the phone.

Do you have stress-producing jobs around your home or office? Find out which jobs are annoying to members of your family or co-workers and see if you can "trade off." You do a job that causes them stress (but doesn't upset you) in exchange for their doing a job that makes you tense (but doesn't bother them). The work gets done and everybody breathes easier.

Are you annoyed by the clutter in your life? Organize your desk, arrange your pots and pans, get the tools out of the drawer and into a tool box where you can find them. If there are clothes in your closet you never wear and regret having bought—give them away. An hour spent removing these causes of stress from your environment can give you a thousand less stressful hours in the future.

These examples could go on forever, but it's *your* list that counts. Take a look at the list you made yesterday. It's time to see how many stresses you can remove from that list simply by removing them physically from your environment.

If you can find just *one* stress on the list and remove it in the next twenty-four hours, you've earned a Feeling Fine point. Give yourself an extra point for each extra stress you eliminate from your list and from your life.

Eating
Pleasures

THE SCS PLAN: SUBSTITUTING

Life is full of choices. Eating is no exception. Each of us has about 100,000 eating occasions in our lifetime, and every time we eat we make choices: between sweet and sour, firm and soft, hot and cold. We can also choose between high calorie count or low, between high nutritional value or low. That's why substituting is such an effective activity if you want eating to become something that's good for your health. The nice thing about it—you don't have to give up the joys of good taste or any of the other real pleasures of food. You may have to give up some of the "target" foods you put on your list two days ago.

It takes remarkably little thought, time, or money to substitute a more nutritious yet just as delicious food for the one you might otherwise select. And, if you make intelligent choices, your body will reward you by keeping your weight constant. If you are overweight you may even drop pounds as you drop one food for another.

Here are some sample substitutions. Try some of them in your own eating program. (The approximate number of calories you'll save is given in parentheses.)

Breakfast
6 ounces of tomato juice for 6 ounces of orange
    juice (save 60)
Poached or soft-boiled eggs for scrambled (save
    15 per egg)
1 slice of whole wheat or rye bread for a corn
    muffin (save 65)

1 cup of puffed wheat for 1 cup of wheat flakes
   (save 40)
Half a grapefruit for a banana (save 70)
8 ounces of buttermilk or skim milk for 8 ounces
   of whole milk (save 55)

Lunch
4 ounces of plain yogurt or cottage cheese for 4
   ounces of sour cream (save 130-140)
8 ounces of orange juice for a chocolate milk
   shake (save 205)
8 ounces of water for 8 ounces of soft drinks
   (save 100)
8 ounces of tomato juice for 8 ounces of Coke or
   Pepsi (save 50-60)
8 ounces of chicken or beef bouillon for 8 ounces
   of any cream soup (save 50-80)
1 tomato for half an avocado (save 150)
7 ounces of water-packed tuna for 7 ounces of
   oil-packed tuna (save 235)
3½ ounces of tuna salad for a hamburger (save
   115)
3 pieces of melba toast for a pan roll (save 55)

Dinner
4 ounces of coleslaw for 4 ounces of potato salad
   (save 70)
4 ounces of cooked carrots or zucchini for 4
   ounces of peas (save 45)
1 medium baked potato (plain) for 8 French fries
   (save 50)
Vegetables with margarine and herbs instead of
   cream sauce (save 50)
3 ounces of broiled chicken for 3 ounces of broiled
   sirloin (save 225)
3 ounces of broiled sole for a 3-ounce pork chop
   (save 245)

4 ounces of meatless spaghetti sauce for 4 ounces
with meat (save 35)

A pear for a piece of cake (save 350)

An apple and 1 ounce of cheddar cheese for 6
ounces of vanilla ice cream (save 105)

4 ounces of canned peaches packed in natural
juice for 4 ounces packed in syrup (save 35)

You can use any of the published calorie lists to
work out your own substitution program. Concentrate
especially on substituting for your "target" foods and
earn a Feeling Fine point whenever you do.

Body Pleasures

MUTUAL MASSAGE: SHARING THE FUN

If you think yesterday's self-massage exercises
were fun, you're in for a real treat. Today's program is
even better.

How do you make it better? There's only one
way. Get someone else to do it.

Your massage partner can be anyone—spouse,
friend, child, or relative—because mutual massage is not
necessarily sexual. Massage is *sensual* (in the true sense of
the word) in that it makes us aware of our bodies. It can
be erotic, but it can also be restful, invigorating, or just
plain pleasurable, depending on the mood and the pace.

Some people say the hardest part is asking
someone to help them. You can break the ice by offering

to massage your partner first. Once you get a partner, here are some ways to make the experience pleasing.

1. Get comfortable with your environment. Low lighting, a quiet room, some music playing, a comfortable temperature in which the exposed body is at ease—all will enhance the mutually relaxing and pleasant feeling of the massage.

2. Remember that what you are massaging is not inanimate. It's human. It's friendly. So when you are on the giving end, enjoy the feeling that is coming through your hands. Ask your partner for verbal responses so that you can learn exactly what feels best. If you hit a point where your partner feels a particular pleasure, continue to massage that area for a moment before moving on. Pay attention to your own responses, too. If you get tired, stop and let your partner do the massaging for a while.

3. Try some body oil. Many drugstores sell massage oils, or you can use olive oil (as in the olden days), baby oil, or even vegetable oil. If you really want to go all out, warm the oil before you put it on the body, to increase the pleasant sensations.

4. Massage easily and gently, with a light pressure or kneading action. Do it continuously, working slowly, smoothly, evenly over the surfaces of the body.

5. Massage from more than one position. This will prevent the discomfort that comes from sitting or kneeling in one place and will also affect the kinds of sensations you receive from your partner.

6. Don't massage infected or inflamed areas. If your partner feels pain, move to another area. All the cautions mentioned for self-massage apply to mutual massage as well.

The variations and refinements of massage are almost without number. Anyone who is fortunate enough to have a partner who also enjoys massage has found a source of Feeling Fine that never diminishes.

Ask your partner to lie down on a comfortable, firm surface. A heavy blanket, a thick rug, or some pillows on the floor should provide satisfactory cushioning. If you have never given a massage, have your partner read the instructions aloud as you work.

BACK MASSAGE ONE

1. Your partner is lying face down, legs together. Straddle your partner's thighs and place your fingers on either side of the body at the base of the spine, but not directly on the spine.

2. With a gentle, circular motion slowly move the flesh on your partner's back up toward the shoulders. Lean forward as you work to add the pressure of your body.

3. When you reach the base of the neck, continue the motion outward toward the shoulders and then down each side of the back.

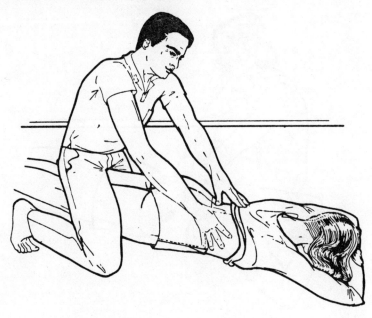

4. When you reach the waist, bring your hands together once more and begin the great circle over again.

BACK MASSAGE TWO

1. Your partner is still lying face down. Sit to the right of your partner at shoulder level and reach across the body, placing one hand on the waist and the other close to it.

2. Keep your hands flat and, alternating their movements, move the flesh inward toward the edge of the spine.

3. Slowly move your hands up from your partner's waist until they reach under the arm.

4. As one hand completes the last stroke under the arm, the other should begin at the waist again.

5. Repeat the process, sitting on your partner's left side.

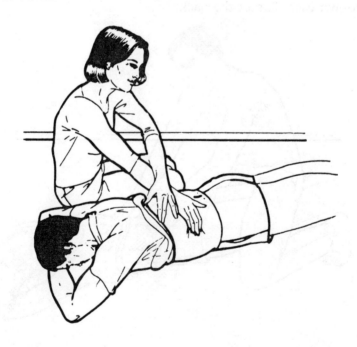

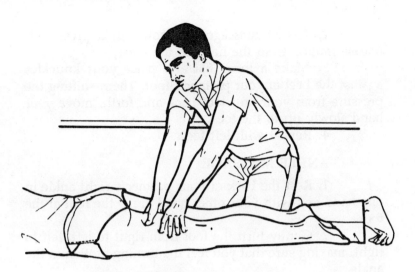

LEG MASSAGE

1. Your partner is lying face down. Sit at your partner's feet in any position that is comfortable for you. You may well want to adjust your position a few times during this massage.

2. Start with your partner's right leg, placing one hand across the ankle and the other just above it, with your fingers facing in opposite directions.

3. Slowly move your hands up the leg toward the knee, applying a gentle, squeezing motion to the flesh on either side of the leg with your fingers and thumbs. As you move up, your body will bend over the leg more and more.

4. When you come to the top of the thigh, move down toward the ankle again.

5. Repeat the process on the left leg.

FOOT MASSAGE

1. With both hands, hold your partner's right foot in your lap with your thumbs on the top of the foot and your fingers on the sole.

2. Gently massage the foot with a press-and-release motion from the heels to the toes.

3. Make a loose fist and place your knuckles against the heel of your partner's foot. Then, shifting the pressure from your knuckles back and forth, move your hand slowly up to the toes.

4. Repeat with left foot.

ANKLE MASSAGE

1. Rest the back of your partner's right ankle in one hand and with your other hand grasp the foot at the toes.

2. Gently turn the foot from right to left, left to right, making sure that you feel the turning motion in the ankle.

3. Repeat with the left ankle.

ARM MASSAGE

1. Your partner is lying face up. Gently grasp your partner's right arm near the armpit, with your thumb on the inside and your fingers on the outside of the arm.

2. With your fingers, slowly and lightly knead down from the upper arm to the forearm and finally to the hand.

3. Work the inside of the hand by using your thumb.

4. Grasp your partner's hand and knead the fingers gently with your fingers.

5. Repeat the procedure with the left arm and hand.

SHOULDER MASSAGE

1. Your partner is lying face down. Place your hands on each side of your partner's neck, fingers close together.

2. Slowly massage your way out across the shoulder muscle. Knead the shoulders, working your fingers back toward the neck.

3. Repeat several times, or until your partner tells you that the muscles feel relaxed.

Give yourself (and your partner) a point for the pleasure of mutual massage.

FEELING FINE POINTS
(Choose one or more from each category.)

GROWING PLEASURES

☐ **Appreciating someone**

☐ Saying no to someone, saying yes to yourself

UNSTRESSING PLEASURES

☐ **Removing a cause of stress**

☐ Finding other causes of stress

EATING PLEASURES

☐ **Substituting few calories for many**

☐ Staying away from your target foods

BODY PLEASURES

☐ **Massaging someone else**

☐ Massaging yourself

DAY 4

Growing Pleasures

REACHING OUT WITH AFFECTION

"Say it with flowers!"

It's the slogan of the florists all over America. It's also a living, blooming testimonial to the fact that most of us no longer can say it with words.

What can't we say with words? Affection.

"I love you."

"I really like you."

"I miss you."

"You mean so much to me."

When is the last time you said something like that to someone? I mean, *really* said it from inside you?

A hundred million dollar greeting card industry has developed because most of us can no longer express affection for each other in our own words. Instead we go to the stationery store and let someone else say it for us. It's easier. Besides, it's safer that way. You haven't stuck your neck out. You haven't really committed yourself. If you are ignored—or worse, rejected—you can always say, "Well, it was only a card." After all, *you* didn't write it.

Yesterday I asked you to reach out to someone with appreciation—with a compliment. That shouldn't have been too hard to do because you really didn't expose any of *yourself* when you did it. Today I want you to reach out to someone again—this time, with affection.

Today's exercise involves feeling. It involves commitment. It also involves joy. It will leave you feeling good—because it's impossible to feel bad when you're telling someone how much you like them.

I'm not going to say any more about it. If you'd like to discover the real pleasure that awaits you in this activity, you're just going to have to do it yourself. Now.

• Find your husband and—no matter where he is or who is watching—tell him you're crazy about him.

• Find your wife and—no matter what she's doing—tell her you love her dearly.

• Find your children and hug them. While you're squeezing, tell them how much you love them.

• Phone a friend. Say, "I miss you."

• Call a co-worker. Say, "I really like you." Is the phone busy? Try again. No answer? Write a note. But do it in your own hand and with your own words.

Is it hard to say the words? Everyone has trouble. Start slowly. Hold a hand. Give a hug. A kiss. But say it. Get some affection right out in the open. You'll feel fine every time you do.

Unstressing Pleasures

REMOVING YOURSELF FROM THE STRESS

It's impossible to remove *all* stress from your environment. That's why sometimes you've got to remove *yourself*. That may sound extremely difficult when what's causing you stress is your job or your spouse. But it's not impossible, and you don't have to quit your job or get a divorce to do it. You just have to learn how to "slip away" for awhile.

There are two ways to slip away: physically and mentally. In a few days we'll be talking about mental trips (the stress-reducing kind). Today, however, we'll concentrate on using your legs to move away from stress.

Some people say the most stressful parts of any working day are coffee breaks and lunchtime. That's when the gossip gets going and the dirt starts flying. That's also when the smart ones start walking. To the park. To the museum. To the parking lot. To solitude. To fresh air and freedom.

Give it a try. Skip the usual coffee break and take a walk around the block. Skip the blue-plate special in the cafeteria and try the brown-bag special in the park.

Even stress-producing situations between husbands and wives can sometimes be relieved by taking a short walk, going bowling with friends, or seeing a movie (alone)—and then returning to face the problem with a lower tension level. Don't be ashamed to take some time away from each other; it can be good for the partnership.

You can remove yourself from all kinds of stressful situations. For example:

• Does being made to wait for something make you angry? Avoid those situations. Shop during off hours, go to a matinée at the movies, eat earlier or later at a restaurant.

• Do you get tense in your doctor's waiting room? Call ahead to make sure you'll be seen on schedule or tell the nurse you'll wait in the coffee shop. Ask her to call you when the doctor is ready.

• Do crowded discount stores give you the creeps? Give the stores a wide berth. You may have to pay a little more for the things you buy, but you'll end up paying a little less to the doctor and the druggist.

Let's get back to your stress list. Are there some environments that come up again and again as triggers for stress? Which ones can you eliminate from your list? Which ones can you eliminate from your life? Move yourself out of a stressful environment and give yourself a point for Feeling Fine.

Eating Pleasures

THE SCS PLAN: CUTTING

Can't believe you ate the whole thing? Then it's time to put a new word into your eating life: cutting.

I mean cutting *back*, not *out*. You don't have to completely give up all your old favorite dishes. You do have to reduce the size of the portions you normally eat, especially the portions of the "target" foods you identified three days ago.

Here's how cutting works (approximate calorie savings are given in parentheses):

Breakfast

1 soft-boiled egg instead of 2 (save 80)

2 slices of bacon instead of 4 (save 45)

1 slice of bread, 1 pat of margarine instead of 2 slices, 2 pats (save 130)

1 tablespoon of peanut butter instead of 3 (save 190)

1 spoonful of honey instead of 3 of jam (save 105)

Half a teaspoon of sugar in your coffee instead of 1 (save 8)

Half the usual amount of cream in your coffee (save up to 50)

Lunch

A cup of chicken noodle soup instead of a bowl (save 50)

A regular MacDonald's hamburger instead of a Big Mac (save 310)

Half a cup of chili instead of a full cup (save 150)

1 burrito instead of 2 (save 50)

2 pieces of pizza instead of 3 (save 130)

3 ounces of luncheon meat instead of 4 (save 50)

Dinner

Meat sautéed in 1 tablespoon of oil instead of 2 (save 125)

1 tablespoon of French dressing instead of 3 (save 65)

Half a cup of rice instead of a full cup (save 100)

3 ounces of meat loaf instead of 6 (save 300)

4 ounces of round steak instead of 8 (save 260)

¾ cup of spaghetti with meat sauce instead of 1½ cups (save 330)

Not everything can be cut in half, but any food can be cut back to some degree. A few tricks can help you do this without making you feel deprived. For example:

1. Use juice glasses instead of regular-sized ones for your drinks.

2. Use salad or dessert plates instead of dinner-sized plates. The same portion makes a fuller plate.

3. Cut meat and bread into thinner slices. Serve the same number of slices.

4. Order one main dish and split it with a friend when you eat out. Half the calories, half the price.

5. Buy a small box of popcorn when you go to the movies—if you *must* have popcorn!

Work especially hard on your "target" foods, but for every cut you make in any food portion today give yourself a Feeling Fine point. Keep it up for the rest of your life and you won't have to worry about your weight. Your point total will grow, but your waistline won't.

Body Pleasures

TAKE A DEEP BREATH

The advertising agencies have made breathing a social disease. They sell you mouthwash, gargles, sprays, and mints so your breath will smell good to others. They want you to believe that all that counts is what you exhale.

Take it from me—*how* you breathe is far more important. It's time to stop breathing to please others and start breathing to pleasure yourself.

You breathe about 23,000 times every day. Do you enjoy it? Do you even notice it? Most people don't —until something goes wrong and they can't breathe normally. By that time it's too late.

Your breathing will often mirror not only your physical condition but your emotional state as well. When you are at peace with yourself and the world around you, your breathing will be slow, deep, and regular. When you are upset or stressed, your breathing rate will accelerate and its rhythm will become erratic. If the stress is great enough, you may suffer an attack of hyperventilation. Then, even though your lungs are taking in far more oxygen than your body requires, your lips and fingertips will become numb, you will become dizzy, and you will feel as though you are choking for air.

With training you can reverse the process. You can actually use your breathing to quiet your mind, ease your stress, and relax your body. This is one of the great benefits of having your breathing under your control. For thousands of years, the Indian Yogis have used breathing control this way. Today, by trying a few of the simplest breathing exercises, you'll experience some of these benefits. Before we start the exercises, here are a few tips to help you obtain the maximum pleasure and effect.

1. Do the exercises in a quiet room. Close the door. Take the phone off the hook. Give full attention to the sounds, sensations, and feeling of your breathing.

2. Sit comfortably in a chair with your arms on your lap or at your sides.

3. Don't let anything restrict your breathing. Loosen your tie and belt, unfasten your bra, unbutton your shirt.

4. Always breathe in through your nose and out through your mouth.

5. When you inhale, concentrate on expanding your ribs and pushing your abdomen out. When you exhale, pull the abdomen in. This is the opposite of the natural tendency to suck in your abdomen when you inhale. Try it.

Now, here are the three breathing exercises.

EXERCISE ONE

1. Exhale comfortably. Don't exaggerate trying to empty yourself of all air, but do pull your abdomen fully in.

2. Inhale rapidly. Take as much air into your chest as you can within 2 seconds.

3. Then take in even more by expanding your abdomen quickly. Try to fill the entire rib cage and abdomen, not just the upper part of your chest, with air.

4. Draw your abdomen in forcibly, pushing the accumulated air out through your mouth.

5. Repeat the process 10 times.

EXERCISE TWO

1. Start as in Exercise One, but inhale more slowly—extend the period of time over which you are drawing in the air to 5 seconds.

2. Hold your breath for 5 seconds. (Until you are used to deep breathing you may not be able to extend your inhalation to 5 seconds. Your ability to do so will grow as you repeat the exercise.)

3. Exhale slowly until your lungs are empty.

4. Repeat 5 times.

EXERCISE THREE

1. With a finger, press your left nostril so that the passage is closed. While counting slowly to 4, draw a deep breath through your right nostril.

2. Close your right nostril with another finger. Hold your breath for 4 seconds.

3. Release your finger from the left nostril and exhale over a period of 4 seconds.

4. Reverse the process, breathing in through the left nostril and exhaling through the right.

5. Repeat the exercise until you have inhaled and exhaled 5 times with each nostril.

Give yourself a point for using your breathing to help you feel fine.

FEELING FINE POINTS
(Choose one or more from each category.)

GROWING PLEASURES
☐ **Saying I love you/I like you**
☐ Appreciating someone
UNSTRESSING PLEASURES
☐ **Removing yourself from stress**
☐ Removing another cause of stress
EATING PLEASURES
☐ **Cutting calories from your diet**
☐ Staying away from your target foods
BODY PLEASURES
☐ **Breathing deeply**
☐ Giving someone else a massage

DAY 5

Growing Pleasures

TIME ALONE

Chores at home. Duties at the office. Problems touching on every aspect of your life. Responsibilities to friends and family. Commitments to the world.

Like a rapidly advancing tide they begin to accumulate in the morning and, as the hours go by, swell and rise to engulf the entire day. Faced by all the "must do's" that overrun your life, how often do you take a little time out just to "be"?

You haven't got time for that, you say. You have too many important things to take care of.

I used to feel that way. Then one day I got sick and couldn't fulfill any of my commitments. That's what it took to make me realize that *I* was the most important thing to take care of. I learned that you don't have to be *doing* something to be doing something for *yourself*.

I learned the simple pleasure that can be gained from lying quietly on the grass for five minutes, even though someone thought I should be mowing it.

I learned the great joy that comes from sitting quietly in my favorite chair for ten minutes, even though there were letters to be answered.

I learned the tremendous peace that can be gained from watching the clouds in the sky and the leaves in the breeze, even though there were tasks to be done.

I learned how to turn off my "doing" world for my "being" world, and I discovered a whole new world of pleasure.

But I had to get sick before I learned that lesson. Don't let that happen to you.

I can't tell you how to spend those five or ten minutes away from your chores. Everyone will use that small break in different ways on different days. If you choose to think about yourself, fine. If the world around you is what occupies your mind, that's fine, too. Whatever you're feeling at the time, relax and let it happen. Just don't *do* anything to spoil it. Enjoy the luxury of simply experiencing what you're feeling at that quiet moment of being alone.

Today's exercise is really simple: take five or ten minutes out of your day to do nothing. No work. No problem solving. No guilt. Just the pure pleasure of a few serene moments alone.

Are you concerned about how you'll find the time? Here are some tricks to help you:

1. If things are too hectic at home or at work, take five or ten minutes alone *before* you get there. If you drive, pull off to the side of the road for your reflection-pause. If you use public transportation, get off one stop early and take a five-minute walk.

2. Skip the usual coffee break at work or use part of your lunch hour. Spend the time alone.

3. If you'd rather do your thinking in the comfort of your home, reserve a few minutes for yourself at a regular time—just before dinner, just after dinner, or right after the children go to bed. Once your family is in the habit of respecting your time alone you'll discover that something you thought you could never find—five minutes alone—was there all the time.

4. If there still isn't enough time in the day, get up five minutes earlier. It's worth the loss of sleep.

No matter when you do it, sit quietly and feel the moment. Let whatever you are experiencing be felt, and let that feeling fill you completely. Then give yourself a Feeling Fine point for experiencing the pleasure of time alone.

Unstressing Pleasures

RETURNING STRESS TO ITS RIGHTFUL OWNER

Have you ever noticed that some of your stress is really someone else's problem? Why do they have to give it to you?

> Like the husband who constantly invites business associates home for dinner and expects his wife to take care of it on short notice.
> Or the wife who's on the board of eleven charitable organizations and expects her husband to be at every fund-raising event.
> The child who runs up huge phone bills and expects his parents to pay them.
> The boss who makes unreasonable commitments to customers and expects his employees to work weekends to meet them.
> Demanding relatives and friends who consistently burden you with their problems and expect you to come up with solutions.

The list goes on and on. *If you let it.* It stops the moment you draw the line. That's what today's activity is all about—drawing the line.

Don't get me wrong. Certainly there's a time for sympathy. There's a time for involvement. There's a time to help others. After all, having a meaningful relationship with someone does carry obligations and responsibilities along with it. But sometimes the person making the request won't have a reasonable answer if you inquire directly, "Why are you asking me to do this?" There's no better question than that to keep someone from coming back again later with the same unjustified demands.

Today start setting limits on the amount of stress you let other people lay on you. It's not hard to do. Here are a few ideas that will help you return some of your stress to its rightful owner.

Be direct. Don't beat around the bush. When someone is trying to lay their difficulties on you, all you have to say is, "That's your problem, not mine. You take care of it." You don't have to be mean or rude but you must be direct. Otherwise you'll find yourself apologizing for not making their stress yours.

Be definite. If you don't want to do something, say so clearly: "No, I will not get involved. Not under any condition." A statement like that leaves little room for negotiations. You don't want to leave any room.

Be honest. Returning stress to its rightful owner does not mean ducking your own work or avoiding unpleasant tasks. Try to distinguish those problems which are really yours and take care of them without complaining. In the long run that's the least stressful thing you can do for yourself, not to mention what you'll be doing for others.

Be quick. Don't waste any time. Right now take a look at your list of stresses. How many of them are someone else's? How will you return them? When will you start?

Prepare yourself to start right away by reviewing "The 'No' That Says 'Yes' " in Day 2 of Growing Pleasures. Then give yourself a Feeling Fine point for every stress you return to its rightful owner.

Eating Pleasures

THE SCS PLAN: SKIPPING

One of my favorite cartoons shows a doctor telling his overweight patient, "I want you to skip eating three meals a day; you're getting enough between meals."

Which brings me to the subject of skipping, the simplest technique of all.

All you have to do is skip foods that are relatively high in concentrated calories for the amount of nutritional value they contain. Chances are we're talking about the "target" foods you put on the list four days ago. Don't forget—you need to drop 10 calories a day if you expect your belt to fit next year. You've got to skip 3,500 calories if you want to lose a pound.

If you'd like some ideas, look at the following list and you'll see how easy it is. (The number in parentheses tells you approximately how many calories you'll save.)

Breakfast
Have the coffee (*with* cream and sugar), skip the
    sweet roll (save 130)
Eat the muffin, skip the jam (save 100)
Have the egg, skip 2 slices of bacon (save 45)

Try an omelet, skip the hash browns (save 235)
Dine on the omelet, skip the cheese (save 160)
Chew the bread, skip the butter (save 100)
Eat the berries, skip the cream and sugar (save
    130)
Devour the blintzes, skip the jam (save 150)
Feast on the waffle, skip the sausages (save 200)

Lunch
Down a burger, skip the fries (save 200)
Have the chicken salad, skip the avocado half
    (save 170)
Consume the sandwich, skip the creamed soup
    (save 140)
Finish the sandwich, skip the potato salad (save
    100)
Eat the steak, skip the onion rings (save 190)
Drink the milk, skip the apple pie (save 330)
Have the taco, skip the beans and rice (save 250)
Enjoy the salad, skip the olives (save 35)
Have the tea, skip the soft drink (save 100)
Have the corn bread, skip the butter (save 200)
Delight in the date nut bread, skip the cream
    cheese (save 105)
Pack away the pudding, skip the whipped
    cream (save 90)

Dinner
Sip the drink, skip the cashews (save 170)
Relish the roast, skip the gravy (save 100)
Finish the chicken, skip the stuffing (save 200)
Eat the vegetable, skip the butter (save 100)
Mash the potato, skip the sour cream (save 90)
Savor the spaghetti, skip the garlic bread (save
    175)
Munch on the asparagus, skip the hollandaise
    (save 50)

Enjoy the soup, skip the crackers (save 45)
Drink the tea, skip the fortune cookie (save 30)
Nibble on the cake, skip the icing (save 70)

Got the idea? Try especially hard to skip your "target" foods, but give yourself a Feeling Fine point for anything high in concentrated calories that you skip today.

Body Pleasures

STEP RIGHT THIS WAY

Robert Frost once said, "I've always walked with my dog. I don't know if it did the dog any good, but it did me."

I don't know how long the dog lived, but Frost lived to be 89. And research studies have shown that people who are active every day live longer than those who are not, even if their activity is something as simple as walking. That's why it's called a "constitutional." Walking is good for the constitution.

It's even good for your weight. Walking one mile at a brisk pace will burn up almost 100 calories. If you held your eating constant but started walking briskly one mile every day, you'd lose ten pounds a year *without dieting*.

If living longer, feeling finer, and losing weight aren't enough to get you off your seat and onto your feet, here's an even better reason: walking is fun! Do you remember how much fun it was to walk around a strange city, taking in all the sights? Can you recall the universal pleasure of childhood—walking in the rain *without an um-*

brella? Can you remember the joy of walking along a beach or through a forest with someone you liked? Those pleasures can be yours again, but you've got to take the first step. You've got to start walking.

There are lots of excuses for why we quit walking. Today none of them is any good. To earn your Feeling Fine point, you're going to have to walk a mile. You don't have the time, you say? You don't know where to start? Here are some tips to help you start walking:

1. Need to take a bus? Don't get on at the nearest stop. Walk past it to the next one. Once on the bus, get off one stop early. Walk the rest of the way to your destination. Or pass your stop and walk back.

2. Driving yourself? Don't look for a parking lot close to where you're going. Pick one six blocks away and use your legs to make up the difference.

3. Going out to lunch? Pick a restaurant half a mile away and walk both ways.

4. Shopping? Park your car as far from the door as possible. Once inside, use the stairs. Leave the elevators and escalators for the infirm.

5. Walk for all your small errands—to the corner mailbox, to the grocer's, to the cleaner's.

6. Walk for pure pleasure. Pick a place you'd really like to explore, go there and walk around. Change the scene of your walk frequently. Anyone can get bored walking the same area over and over. Drive to a good spot if you have to. Ten or fifteen minutes by car will take you to dozens of interesting places to walk, where you can be entertained by sights and sounds which are different from those outside your door. It's not hard to squeeze a one-mile walk into your day.

7. One thing you shouldn't squeeze is your feet. Wear a sturdy pair of comfortable walking shoes with good arches. Never mind the stylish heels or tall platforms when you're out walking. You're not trying to please anyone but yourself.

8. Try "interval walking"—alternating periods of very rapid walking with a normal pace. Do each for a specific distance or period of time.

9. If you want the ultimate in pleasure and you're anywhere near a beach—forget the shoes and walk in the sand. You'll never want to stop.

Whatever shoes you choose, walk your mile and give yourself another Feeling Fine point.

FEELING FINE POINTS
(Choose one or more from each category.)

GROWING PLEASURES

☐ **Taking time alone**

☐ Breaking a taboo

UNSTRESSING PLEASURES

☐ **Returning stress to its rightful owner**

☐ Keeping an eye on your stress target organs

EATING PLEASURES

☐ **Skipping calories**

☐ Substituting calories

BODY PLEASURES

☐ **Walking for pleasure**

☐ Breathing deeply

DAY 6

Growing Pleasures

PURE PLEASURE ON $1 A DAY

In this age of inflation not even a millionaire can afford to live like one. But you don't have to be a millionaire—or even live like one—to feel like a million dollars. You just need to learn how to spend a buck wisely.

Not long after we were married, my wife, Priscilla, and I treated ourselves to a European vacation. That's not an easy thing to do when you're in medical school and your wife is paying the bills out of a secretary's salary. But we decided we had to go, since we were sure that it must be now—or very, very much later. To make sure that we could afford the trip we decided to follow the young traveler's Bible, *Europe on Five Dollars a Day*.

It wasn't always possible to follow the book's advice. After seventy-seven days the tab came to $6.50 per person, per day. Not bad. We learned that we didn't have to stay at the Savoy to enjoy London. A bed-and-breakfast pension near the London Museum gave us a comfortable night's sleep and a good breakfast to boot. In Paris we didn't have to dine at the Tour d'Argent to savor French food. A tiny Left Bank bistro proved to be a first-rate experience.

Many of us have similar experiences when we

are young and forced to live on small budgets. As we grow older and our incomes expand we forget how we used to derive pleasure from life without spending huge amounts of money. We start treating ourselves to expensive meals that make us feel very good—until the bill arrives. We stay in plush hotels and feel like royalty—until the cashier brings us back to reality. We buy big cars loaded with extras and feel great—until we write out the monthly check for the loan payment. But pleasure doesn't have to come with a big bill attached.

Think back to the number of times you have denied yourself something you wanted because it cost more than you planned to spend. Even just a little more. Maybe it was a jar of imported jam that cost 39¢ more than your regular brand, and you didn't buy it for that reason. Maybe it was a bottle of wine in a restaurant that cost a dollar more than the kind you normally order, and you resisted because of that extra dollar. Or maybe it was a somewhat better seat in a theater.

Sometimes we don't spend the dollar for exactly the opposite reason—the thing we want to buy isn't expensive enough.

How often have you decided that a small, spur-of-the-moment gift that you knew a friend would enjoy wasn't "good" enough to give—because it only cost a dollar? How often have you said no to a passing fancy because you knew that your pleasure would just be momentary? How often have you not spent a buck because the purchase was "foolish" and not something you really needed?

I'd call that penny-wise, pleasure-foolish. The Growing Pleasure for today will be to give yourself a present—a dollar bill (or two, if you really feel high-spirited)—and see how much pleasure you can squeeze out of it. This exercise is so much fun, you're going to want to do it every day for the rest of your life.

Want some ideas?
- Treat someone to a cup of coffee.
- Buy a ball or a Frisbee and find someone to throw it with.
- Buy a frame and put a pretty postcard in it.
- Get a photo you're especially fond of blown up.
- Buy a tiny plant or a flower.
- Visit a dime store and buy a gift for less than a buck.
- Buy the absolutely best piece of fruit you can find and eat it slowly.
- Make a *short* long-distance phone call.
- Buy a gadget for your kitchen or tool box.
- Buy a copy of an interesting paperback and give it to a friend.
- Visit a stationer's or art supply store and see what they have that you've always wanted—for under a buck.
- Give the dollar away.

Whatever you choose to do with your dollar, think of it as a present to yourself.

Anytime a dollar stands between you and pleasure, spend the buck and buy yourself another Feeling Fine point.

Unstressing Pleasures

EASING STRESS WITH GUIDED IMAGERY

Dying is the only sure way to remove every single stress from your life. It isn't worth it. There are other ways to stop the toll stress takes on your body.

Guided imagery is one of those ways. Here's how it works.

Your brain contains a collection of nerve cells called the hypothalamus, which controls many of your body's functions. The hypothalamus gathers information (through your senses of sight, touch, hearing, taste, and smell) and uses that information to make your body respond in an appropriate way.

For example, when you smell sizzling bacon on the stove, it's the hypothalamus that orders your salivary glands into action and gets your stomach and intestines growling. When you see a speeding car bearing down on you, it's your hypothalamus that gets the adrenaline surging and the heart pounding so you can jump quickly out of the way.

You don't even need sizzling bacon or a speeding car to trigger the hypothalamus into action. It can respond to *symbolic* stimuli almost as well as to real ones. When you look at a really good picture of roast turkey and cranberry sauce your salivary glands may start working as if the real thing were in front of you. Watch a truly terrifying movie and your heart may pound and your palms sweat as much as if you were actually in real danger.

That's how guided imagery works. Picture a tranquil scene and your hypothalamus will help you become tranquil yourself. Picture a healthy body and you will become healthier in the process. Give your brain some relaxing and healthful pictures to work on and the hypothalamus will "order" a calmer, more relaxed body for you to enjoy.

The kind of relaxation we are trying to teach in guided imagery (and later in the book, with autogenics, meditation, and other techniques) is not the same kind of relaxation we may feel after an evening of TV viewing or an afternoon spent quietly with friends. Those activities, and most of the other things we think of as relaxing (like recreational sports or vacation travel) demand a fairly high degree of physical and mental activity, as we follow the plot of a story, engage in the give-and-take of conversation, hit the ball, or travel from one new place to another.

Guided imagery and the other kinds of relaxation techniques involve turning your attention inward, not outward—quieting the body, not stimulating it. They involve physically and mentally letting go of the tensions that your body and mind have acquired at work and even during your "relaxing" pleasures.

I was first introduced to guided imagery while making a film of relaxation techniques with Dr. David Bresler, a psychologist at UCLA. Our cameraman—who was a pretty tense individual—developed a severe headache. Dr. Bresler used guided imagery to help the cameraman relax and, within minutes, his headache was gone. I don't have headaches, but I often get tense, so I tried guided imagery to see if it would make the tension go away. The results were dramatic. I've used it ever since to make tension disappear in seconds.

Over the next few days you'll learn how to make guided imagery work for you. Here's the basic technique.

1. Find a private place where you won't be interrupted for at least five minutes. Close the door, take the phone off the hook, and ask people to leave you alone.

2. Sit down in a comfortable chair, loosen your clothing, and relax. Don't lie down or you're liable to fall asleep.

3. Close your eyes and take five deep breaths. Breathe in through your nose. Breathe out through your mouth, keeping your lips slightly pursed as you do. Each time you breathe in, silently say to yourself: "I am." Each time you breathe out, say: "relaxed." "I am . . . (breathing in) . . . relaxed . . . (breathing out). I am . . . relaxed."

4. Create a peaceful picture in your mind's eye.

Select the picture from one of the following three scenes:

• A beautiful beach on a tropical isle: Imagine white sand in the hot sun with gently waving palms, deep blue water with gentle waves, fleecy clouds in an azure sky.

• A valley nestled deep between two mountain ranges: Pretend it is spring and the green carpet of the valley is broken only by the brilliant colors of the wildflowers and the reed roofs of cottages far away in the distance. The quiet is penetrated only by the gentle gurgling of a brook and the song of a hundred birds.

• A farm scene during harvest: Imagine that dappled cows are making their way slowly across the valley floor. The sounds of their lowing and the gentle clanging of their bells mingle with the sounds of birds in the air and the wind in the trees.

5. Move yourself into the picture you're imagining. Place yourself in a comfortable position—on the ground, against a tree, even in a chair. In your mind's eye try to hear, see, and feel every detail of the scene as though you were really there. Concentrate as much as you can on details of the scene. Zoom up close on things like leaves and flowers and colors. Try to sense the heat of the sun on your skin or the movement of wind against your hair. Be there—as if you were really there.

6. Spend five minutes on this journey. Then slowly open your eyes and return to the physical world you're in. Don't get up for at least sixty seconds. During that time take note of how you feel. Your body should feel extremely relaxed. Your mind will feel refreshed.

It's time now to take a relaxing trip to the center of your mind's eye. Use guided imagery to get you there and give yourself a Feeling Fine point.

Eating
Pleasures

TRIMMING THE FAT

During the next few days we'll look at some specific nutrients you take into your body and talk about some of the problems these things cause. Obviously we can't discuss everything, but we'll cover those subjects we should be most concerned about. Today let's talk about fats.

Saturated fats play a role in several diseases, particularly disorders of the circulatory system, and they wreak havoc with the waistline. It's not fat in itself that causes all the trouble. It's *too much* fat that does it— especially saturated fat, the kind that comes from animal sources.

There are now some people who claim that all of the disorders caused by excess fat—even atherosclerosis (hardening of the arteries caused by fatty deposits)—can be reversed by cutting the dietary intake of fat way down. Maybe so. The trouble is, the diet they suggest is almost impossible to follow unless you have your own full-time chef or $3,000 a month to pay the tab at one of the "rejuvenation" resorts.

There is an alternative. It's called "trimming the fat." Businesses trim the fat out of their budgets because it's good for the health of the business. You've got to trim the fat out of your diet because it's good for the health of your body.

It's really not hard to trim the fat. Here are some simple tips to help you do it.

1. Eat less meat. Red meat is one of the richest sources of fat. Most of us eat far more meat than we need.

2. If you must eat meat, buy lower grades of beef. Although "prime" or "choice" are supposed to be the preferred cuts, "good" and "standard" grades are leanest. They contain more protein and less fat. They also cost less.

3. Cut all visible fat off your meat and discard it—*before* the meat goes into the broiler, pot, or on the barbecue. After it's cooked, cut off any remaining fat you can still see.

4. Broil your meats. Don't pan-fry them.

5. Cook meat on a rack so the fat will drip away into a pan rather than soak into the meat.

6. Baste meat with water, wine, or tomato juice, not meat drippings.

7. Trim off by skimming off. Cook stew, spaghetti sauce, and soup one day ahead and place in the refrigerator. The fat will congeal on the top so that you can scoop it off and throw it away before you reheat and serve.

8. Brown meats under the broiler, not with oil in a skillet.

9. Eat fewer organ meats (brains, liver, and kidneys). They are chock full of cholesterol.

10. Get in the habit of substituting poultry and fish for meat (but avoid shrimp, which is high in cholesterol).

11. Don't buy prebasted turkeys. The basting is usually done with saturated fats. When you eat poultry, don't eat the skin.

12. Buy water-packed tuna. If you do use oil-packed tuna, squeeze out as much of the oil as possible before preparing it.

13. Be careful with eggs. They contain a lot of cholesterol, (some nutritionists say eggs are okay if boiled or poached, but not if fried).

14. Substitute margarine made with unsaturated

oil for butter. (Read the label—not all "lower-priced spreads" include unsaturated fats.)

15. Switch from whole milk to lowfat or nonfat.
16. Steer clear of ice cream.
17. Avoid butter-based sauces and deep-fried foods.
18. Use unsaturated oils such as corn, soybean, or safflower for salads and cooking.

If you contact the American Heart Association in your city they will gladly send you booklets of ideas and recipes to help you cut saturated fats from your diet.

For each suggestion you carry out, give yourself a Feeling Fine point.

Body Pleasures

IT'S WHAT'S UP BACK THAT COUNTS

In two years of health reporting on television, no single segment has attracted more viewer mail than one show I did on the subject of back problems. Why, I wondered, did that happen?

I suffer from frequent backaches myself, so the answer should have been obvious: a healthy back is the foundation for a healthy body. When your back isn't feeling good, nothing else in your body can feel the way it should.

I got my backaches the hard way. I fractured a vertebra in an accident while riding a motorcycle to work when I was an intern. For years I suffered daily back-aches, an experience I had never known before. I began to view my days in surgery as days of punishment, when before they had always been days of challenge and satisfaction. The challenge became how to get through the schedule of operations without a crushing backache.

Several surgeons suggested I have a back operation. I was too afraid to consider it. Some doctors suggested I change my schedule. I couldn't. Others suggested I change my medical specialty. I wouldn't. Finally, one doctor suggested I change the way I treated my back. His suggestions changed my life.

I learned how to avoid most of my backaches through simple tricks of posture and common sense. The techniques he taught me are good for your back, even if you haven't been knocked off a motorcycle. They're the best way I know to make a bad back feel better and keep a good back feeling fine. Let me share them with you now.

WHEN SITTING

1. Try to keep at least one knee higher than your hips. This, too, automatically gives you the healthiest spinal curve.

2. If you sit at a table, desk, or sewing machine, use a small hassock or stool to prop one or both feet up. Don't stretch out your legs.

3. When driving, sit close to the steering wheel. This forces you to keep one knee higher than your hips.

4. When reading or watching television, use a chair that supports head, neck, and arms. Don't thrust your head forward. Never read or watch television lying down.

WHEN STANDING

1. If you must stand for prolonged periods, try to keep one leg bent slightly. Raising the foot automati-

cally keeps your spinal curvature in its healthiest position and avoids back strain. (Now you understand the reason for a foot rail in bars. It allows people to stand there for a long time without feeling any pain.)

    2. Shift your weight occasionally from one foot to the other.

    3. Position yourself so that you're face to face with your work. When you turn, pivot with your feet before you turn your upper body.

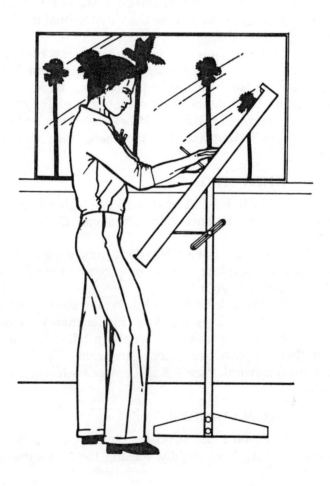

WHEN LEANING, LIFTING, OR REACHING

1. When lifting objects from the floor, keep your back straight. Bend at the hips and knees, never from the waist. Hold heavy objects close to your body.

2. Avoid long reaches. Use a stool. Keep your buttocks tucked in as you reach.

3. When working with tools such as a broom or rake, always hold them close to your body.

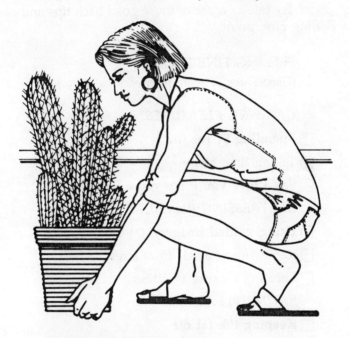

WHEN SLEEPING

1. Ignore the mattress ads, which generally show people sleeping on their front or back. The best posture for sleeping is curled up on your side with your knees flexed. According to Islamic tradition, kings sleep on the right side, wise men on the left, saints on their backs. The devil sleeps on his stomach. I suggest never sleeping on

your stomach or you, too, may eventually feel like the devil. It makes your body sag into the bed and gives your back a painful arch. If you want to be a saint and sleep on your back, place a pillow under your lower legs and feet to give your body added support.

2. Use a firm mattress.

3. Use a low, soft pillow to avoid putting stress on your neck.

Try one or more of these good back tips and earn a Feeling Fine point.

FEELING FINE POINTS
(Choose one or more from each category.)

GROWING PLEASURES

☐ **Spending $1 for fun**

☐ Taking time alone

☐ Say I love you/I like you

UNSTRESSING PLEASURES

☐ **Using guided imagery**

☐ Removing yourself from stress

☐ Locating a cause of stress

EATING PLEASURES

☐ **Keeping the fat off**

☐ Skipping calories

☐ Substituting calories

BODY PLEASURES

☐ **Giving your back some support**

☐ Massaging someone

☐ Keeping your senses alive

DAY 7

Growing Pleasures

GOALS: GETTING TO KNOW YOU

What do you want to be when you grow up?

Too many people spend their whole lives working and never getting where they want to be. Others struggle to get where they want to be, only to find out they don't like it there. What are your goals?

Some people say that it's a waste of time setting goals. Life, they say, is in the hands of fate. They bounce from one thing to another, never thinking about what life may hold in store next. They often complain that somehow life isn't very satisfying, and they never fail to have a good excuse if things don't work out the way they had hoped.

Other people spend their lives trying to achieve goals set for them by someone else—by mothers who want them to be lawyers, fathers who want them to run businesses, wives who want possessions, and husbands who want handmaidens. The result? Law degrees, money, furs, status, a tidy house, and basic dissatisfaction. The things that are often missing are happiness, health, fulfillment, and pleasure.

There are those who set goals early in life and follow them without fail—and without change. For twenty or thirty or forty years they work toward these goals. The times change, the people change, their needs change.

But the goals never change. Long before the age of re-
tirement arrives, the goals don't mean anything any more.
They no longer seem worth the price that has to be paid,
but it's too late.

How can *you* avoid this dissatisfaction?

By looking at yourself as a growing being and by
setting goals for that growth. By accepting responsibility
for your fate and taking time to do something about it. By
recognizing the world as a changing place and allowing
yourself to change with it.

That's what today's exercise is all about. Taking
a look at yourself, your world, and your goals, and giving
yourself the opportunity to change. For today's exercise
forget your age. Forget "where you are" in life. Forget
your past decisions. Forget all restrictions and start with a
clean slate. Right now, if you could start all over again at
this point, WHAT WOULD YOU WANT TO BE WHEN YOU GROW UP?

To earn your Feeling Fine point for the day, all
you've got to do is answer that question—in writing. Get
yourself a large piece of paper and put your goals down
in black and white.

That's not as easy as it sounds. Some people
find when they get down to it that they have very little to
write. That can be upsetting. Some people discover they
have too much to write. That can be confusing. But either
of those alternatives is better than not even trying to
write.

I've written enough already. Now it's your turn
to pick up the pen. Get your paper and put down your
goals for the future. Carry the paper around with you for
the next twenty-four hours. Add a new goal to your list
whenever it comes to mind. Save the paper, because tomorrow we'll be looking more carefully at those goals—
and at your future.

Start the activity now and there's a Feeling Fine
point in your future.

Unstressing Pleasures

A PLACE OF YOUR OWN

If you took the guided-imagery trip with us yesterday you learned that your body can't tell the difference between a relaxing picture in the mind's eye and the real thing. Your body automatically relaxes in either place.

Yesterday you were given a choice of three relaxing scenes to visit, typical relaxing scenes familiar to all of us through pictures. But none of these scenes is likely to be as relaxing for you as the one you pick yourself—from your memories or your dreams. So today you'll take a guided-imagery trip to the most relaxing place in the world for *you*.

It might be a scene from your youth: a farm you visited, a mountain you camped on, a room you grew up in. Maybe it's more recent: your honeymoon spot, a vacation stop, a desert spa, a cabin by a lake. We all have special places in our hearts, places that—for each of us —are the most relaxing and pleasurable spots on earth. (Mine is a snow-covered bowl at Mammoth Mountain.) All you have to do is use guided imagery to move your spot from your heart into your mind's eye, and your body will relax as though you were really there.

That's your activity for today. Pick a place of your own and visit it through guided imagery. Let's review the technique you'll use:

1. Find some privacy. Protect yourself from interruptions.

2. Make yourself comfortable. Sit down in an easy chair and relax.

3. Close your eyes and take five deep breaths. Each time you take a breath silently say the words, "I am relaxed."

4. Draw a picture in your mind's eye of *your* special relaxing spot. Keep your eyes closed and wait until the picture comes into clear focus and vivid color.

5. Put yourself into the picture. Find a comfortable spot and settle into it. Ask yourself to feel as though you really are there. Examine the scene, look for every possible detail. Look for details *in* the details. If there is a stream in the landscape, look at the color of the water. Feel the flow of the current. Look for rocks jutting out of the stream. Study the grass along the banks. Imagine the refreshing coolness of the water.

If you are in the forest, look at the trail you are following, the dead leaves that cover it in spots. Take note of the trees at the trail's edge, the coloring and markings on the bark, the shape of the branches as they curve over the path. Look at wildflowers at the side of the trail, study their petals. Zoom in for details. Pan back for perspective. Relax. Smile. Enjoy.

6. Spend at least five minutes there. Then slowly open your eyes to the physical world you're in. Return to this world slowly, taking sixty seconds to enjoy the sense of relaxation in your body and the pleasure in your mind.

Take this relaxing trip with guided imagery and give yourself another point for Feeling Fine.

Eating Pleasures

FIBER: SLIP ME SOME SKIN

For years it was the food that people couldn't get rid of fast enough. The bakers milled it away. The refiners strained it away. The restaurants peeled it away. And housewives threw it away.

Until Dr. David Reuben wrote a book about it. Now it's the most popular thing in the world next to sex. What is it? You guessed it!

Fiber.

It's the undigestible parts of foods which pass through our digestive system unchanged. The skin of the cucumber, the seed of the eggplant, the rind of the orange, the bran of the wheat.

Fiber fans say it will prevent cancer of the colon and eliminate heart disease. Is that true? No one knows for sure. People who eat fiber-rich foods do seem to have less heart disease, but no one knows whether this is due to the fiber itself or to the fact that fiber-eaters tend to eat fewer animal fats. It is true, however, that people with fiber-rich diets don't suffer much constipation. That alone is a pretty good reason for adding more fiber to your daily food intake.

The fiber enthusiasts say you should eat at least an ounce of fiber a day. People on average diets already eat a quarter ounce a day, so if you're in that category you don't have too far to go. Here's what to do to eat more fiber:

1. Buy whole-grain products. They are much richer in fiber than the refined ones. Use whole grains (cornmeal, wheat, rye, rolled oats, buckwheat) for your breads, pancakes, and cereals.

2. Use brown rice instead of white rice.

3. Eat popcorn (with *very little* butter, of course).

4. Try pumpkin or sunflower seeds and nuts (it's best to buy them with the shells still on). Not too many, though—they're high in calories.

5. Increase the amount of fresh vegetables and fruits you eat. Don't peel them clean and white; eat the skins of such things as cucumbers, eggplants, and apples

whenever possible, since that's where the fiber content is.

6. When you squeeze oranges and other citrus fruits, don't strain the juice. Drink pulp and all.

7. Bran for breakfast is easy—it's readily available in commercial cereals. You can also buy unprocessed miller's bran, which is cheaper but it tastes awful. Miller's bran is easier to take if you mix it into fruit juice or yogurt, sprinkle it on soups, or bake it into bread.

8. Read the labels on the products you buy to be sure you're getting fiber. If it says only "wheat flour," the fiber has been removed. It must say "100 percent *whole grain.*"

Give yourself a Feeling Fine point every time you put a high-fiber food into a meal.

Body Pleasures

LIMBERING UP TO SAVE YOUR NECK

Would you like to be able to move as easily at the age of 80 as you did at 8? This flexibility is yours for the asking or, better yet, for the limbering.

Take a moment to try a few simple motions.

1. Bring your chin down to your chest.

2. Turn your head as far to the right as it will go. Now to the left.

3. Stand up with your right hand dangling at your side. Make a sweeping circle with your arm. Repeat with your left arm.

4. With your arms straight out in front of you at shoulder height, raise your left leg in front of you as high

as it will go, and return. Do the same with your right leg.

5. Keeping your back straight, bend at the knees and go all the way down, as if you were picking something up from the floor. Return to a standing position.

Were your movements fluid and flexible? Did you experience any stiffness, pain, or crackling sounds? Or are you still down on your knees?

Remember how you fared, because in the next four days we're going to work on loosening up your body joints and increasing your ability to move, bend, turn, look, kick, and lift.

Part of Feeling Fine is being able to turn your neck around to say hello to a friend in back of you without feeling any pain. It is bending over to put on your shoes and being able to get back up again afterward.

As we grow older, many of us begin to experience difficulties in moving our limbs. We attribute it to arthritis, bursitis, rheumatism, or just old age. Frequently it's none of these. It happens because we've given up using our joints, and joints which aren't moved soon can't move.

In addition, aches and pains may keep us from moving joints as far as we should because it hurts when we do. So we only move the joints part way for awhile, and soon we can't move them all the way. Little by little, we give up part of the possible range of our joints until we have no range at all. Then we're not only in pain, we're stuck!

It's a vicious circle you should never get into. And the limbering exercises you'll see in a moment will keep it from starting. If you are already feeling those aches and pains, the limbering exercises will go a long way toward bringing you back to the movement you've given up.

Limbering up is important, so it's a good idea to pick a regular time in which to practice. Morning is best because it loosens you up for the rest of the day. (A shower is a superb place to begin when you're feeling stiff. Limbering up in warm water aids the joint movements.) If morning is not convenient, find another time: coffee-break time, lunchtime, before going to bed. A few minutes is all you need. The payoff lasts a lifetime.

If a solid chunk of time is not possible, break up the exercise: do one joint at a time. Limber your knees in the morning, your neck at coffee time, your elbows while watching television. If you take several one-minute limbering breaks for each day we've mapped out, your whole body will thank you.

All exercises should be done slowly and evenly. Make no sharp, jerky, rapid movements. Begin with the recommended number of repetitions, decreasing or increasing as you feel the need. If it hurts, do not push a joint any further. But don't hold back because you think a joint *may* hurt. That's the easiest way to lose function. Just go slowly.

One of the joints many people allow to deteriorate first is the neck joint. Today, therefore, we have three exercises to save your neck. Let's begin.

NECK-SAVER ONE

1. Bend your head all the way back as far as it will comfortably go.

2. Bring your head forward as far as it will go, until your chin presses against your chest.

3. Repeat the front-back cycle 10 times.

NECK-SAVER TWO

1. Begin with your chin on your chest.

2. Roll your head in a continuous circle all the way around until you have circled it from right shoulder to your back to your left shoulder and back to the chest again.

3. Rotate 5 times to the right. Then rotate to the left 5 times.

NECK-SAVER THREE

1. Turn your head to the right, peering backward over your shoulder as far as you can. Return your head to the front.
2. Repeat 5 times.
3. Repeat the process over your left shoulder.

Give yourself a Feeling Fine point for saving your neck today.

FEELING FINE POINTS
(Choose one or more from each category.)

GROWING PLEASURES

☐ **Setting goals**

☐ Appreciating someone

☐ Saying no to someone, saying yes to yourself

UNSTRESSING PLEASURES

☐ **Finding a place of your own**

☐ Returning stress to its rightful owner

☐ Removing yourself from stress

EATING PLEASURES

☐ **Putting fiber in your diet**

☐ Trimming the fat

☐ Pursuing thin calories

BODY PLEASURES

☐ **Saving your neck**

☐ Giving your back some support

☐ Enjoying self-massage

DAY 8

Growing
Pleasures

GOALS: GAINING YOUR BALANCE

Let me guess about the goals you wrote down
yesterday. When you grow up you want to be:
Happy?
Healthy?
Well-adjusted?
You didn't forget those things, did you? Almost
everyone does. People tend to write goals for careers,
goals for income, goals for possessions—but they neglect
goals for themselves. Why? Because in the striving world
in which we live it's the material things that most people
associate with success.

Most people, but not the people who are really
successful at living. They never forget the other things.
They've learned that wealth isn't worth it if it is gained at
the expense of health. Power isn't worth it if it is pur-
chased at the cost of having friends. And fame isn't
worth it at the expense of constant stress. What's their
secret for real success?

Balance. These people have gotten balance in
their living. Ask for their list of goals and you'll find
categories like Health, Pleasure, Personal Growth, and
Relationships with Others. Sure there'll be categories for
Work and Money, too. But by and large their goals for
living will be spread among many categories.

How about you? Are your goals in balance?

It's not hard to find out. All you have to do is review the goals you wrote down yesterday. Check them against the following categories:

☐ Health   ☐ Career, Work
☐ Pleasure   ☐ Financial
☐ Relationships   ☐ Personal
   with Others   Growth

Now take a good look at the boxes. Could you put at least one mark in every one? If so, maybe your goals are already in pretty fair balance.

Are there marks in only one, two, or three of the boxes? Then there's more for you to do today. Your goal for today will be to write at least one goal for each category. Here are some tips to make your goal writing a little easier.

1. *Don't be afraid to dream.* There's no need at this point to reject an idea just because it doesn't seem practical. Your impractical idea may end up giving you a clue about something else that is more practical—and just as desirable.

2. *Use your past.* Reflect on past pleasures and past successes. Have you forgotten some real sources of satisfaction? Maybe it's time to try them again. Think about things that didn't work well, too. Maybe now the time is right to learn from the mistakes of the past. You don't have to be discouraged by them. Use the lessons from these experiences to help you set new goals.

3. *Learn from others.* Make a list of people you admire, then figure out specifically what it is about them you would like for yourself. Don't think about their accomplishments (that may inhibit you) but rather about their personal characteristics that you admire. Certainly don't limit your list to the rich or the famous. Think about the people in your life who seem to have balance.

4. *Ask for help.* Sometimes it's hard to sort these things out when you're talking to yourself. It may be helpful to talk to others. Describe your goals to them. Let them ask questions and push you to clarify what you really want from life. The more you're able to reflect aloud about your own goals, the easier it will be to know them and call them your own.

One word of caution, however. Don't let others judge your goals and talk you into adopting theirs. Talking to others about your goals is good only if it helps you hear yourself. If all you hear is the other person, it's time to talk about something else.

Balance your goals by filling in the categories you've neglected and give yourself another Feeling Fine point.

Unstressing Pleasures

FINDING A FRIEND WITH GUIDED IMAGERY

Thanks to guided imagery you never have to be alone again. Yesterday you used guided imagery to create a relaxing place. Today you'll use it to populate your restful spot with a companion for yourself. You'll learn how to use your mind's eye to create a creature with a mind of its own.

I know it sounds wacky, but it really works. If you find yourself a little doubtful, you're in good company. Once at a medical dinner I was discussing guided imagery with a group at my table, and one of the doctors dismissed it with a single word: "Absurd!" I asked him to try the technique right there at the dinner table. He agreed. Within seconds, he was relaxing, his mind back on a farm he remembered from his boyhood.

"What is the first animal you see?" I asked.

"A deer," he said.

"Boy or girl?"

"How am I supposed to know that?"

"Ask," I suggested.

There was silence. "Boy," he said.

"And what is its name?"

"Bambi," he finally answered. And then his face reddened.

The doctor felt he had been made a fool. But his embarrassment vanished as we discussed his experience. What's wrong with visualizing a deer named Bambi?

There's nothing wrong with it. Not if it gives you pleasure. Certainly not if it gives you company. Soon we'll be showing you how to use the creature in your special place for all of those things and more. For now, however, we'll concentrate only on helping you to bring that creature into focus. Today all you have to do to earn a point is find your companion and make a friend. Here's how you do it.

1. In your mind's eye return to your special relaxing place. Make the picture as vivid as you can and put yourself into it, as you did before.

2. Slowly look around your relaxing scene until you spot a living creature. Don't be surprised by what you find. It could be anything from a zebra to a whale. (I found a rabbit when I first looked. Now *he's* there every time *I* am.)

3. Move in closer on the creature. Ask it to move a little closer to you. (Bear with me; I haven't lost my senses. Ask the creature to move closer and it will.)

4. Now that the creature is up close, it's time for the two of you to get acquainted. This may make you feel a little silly, but don't let that keep you from doing it. Talk to your creature. Tell it your name. Ask *its* name. Believe it or not, you'll get an answer. (My rabbit creature is named Corky. Don't ask me where that name came from. He also said he was a boy.)

5. Now talk with your creature. Any topic will do. When you and your creature have said all there is to say, it's time to return to *this* world again. Say goodbye and promise you'll return again. Then slowly open your eyes.

What's the point of all this conversation with creatures? By using guided imagery to talk to an imaginary creature you are learning how to use the visual powers of your brain. For today, the point is pleasure and amusement. Make a friend with the creature in your mind's eye and you'll never have to be lonely again. In days to come we'll show you how to use this technique for pain relief and problem solving.

But all you have to do for now is find your friend and you've earned another Feeling Fine point.

Eating Pleasures

SUGAR: CUT OUT THE SWEET TALK

The average American eats about 150 pounds of sugar a year, but the picture is not as sweet as it sounds. The reward for eating all that sugar will be a mouthful of cavities and an extra measure of fat.

Sugar provides fertile breeding ground for bacteria that propagate and eat away at your teeth. It also makes you obese, since it's easily converted into fat in the body.

Sometimes sugar is easy to see—the white granules in the sugar bowl. But you'd better be aware that even when you can't see it, you're getting lots of invisible sugar when you eat cookies, candy bars, and many of the processed foods you buy. It's not just in the heavy syrup around the canned fruit, but also in breakfast cereals, breads, soups, bologna, deviled ham, cheese, canned vegetables such as peas, corn, and tomatoes, frozen vegetables, yogurt, mayonnaise, mustard.

There's only one way to find the "invisible" sugar.

Read the ingredient labels on the food you buy. By law, ingredients must be listed in order of quantity. If the word "sugar" is high on the list, you are buying a lot of it.

Keep in mind that manufacturers do not always adhere to the spirit of the ingredient-disclosure law. Rather than admit the embarrassing fact that their products are loaded with sugar, cereal makers, for instance, may put different *kinds* of sugars into their product. That allows them to break up their ingredient list so that it looks like you're getting less sugar. Their list may look like this: gluc-*ose*, wheat, sucr-*ose*, other parts of wheat, fruct-*ose*, iron, *corn syrup*, etc. Though the list sounds nutritionally imposing, all these *-ose* words mean only that the word "sugar" should head the list.

Most of us love sugar because we have been conditioned since infancy by the food industry to want it. It's even put into baby food. Not to please the baby but to please the mother who samples her infant's food. The result is that, very early, children get conditioned to the sweet life.

You can stop that. If you have youngsters, train them early to do without gobs of sugar. Make your own baby food. Don't buy cookies and cakes and candies. The kids won't appreciate it now, but they'll thank you later. When we banned cookies and candies from our home (so I could lose weight) my three kids complained at first. After a while there were still no cookies and finally no complaints. They had learned to do without the sugar.

You can do the same. You'll be surprised how good coffee or tea can be once you get used to the taste of no sugar at all.

Here are some steps you can take to decrease your intake of refined sugar.

1. Eat fruits fresh or frozen, not canned in sugary syrup.

2. If you want to sweeten your cereal, substitute raisins, sliced bananas, strawberries, or other fruit. You'll end up eating less sugar. You'll also find that if you use a little cinnamon on your cereal you won't miss the sugar so much.

3. Starting now, cut in half the amount of sugar you add to foods. Start with your coffee or tea. Continue with your grapefruit and cereal. Keep cutting the amount of sugar every time, and before long you won't need any.

You can't do it in a day or two. Do it gradually. But every time you cut your sugar portion give yourself a Feeling Fine point.

Body Pleasures

LIMBERING UP TO SAVE YOUR SHOULDERS

One elderly Hollywood personality amused everyone at a dinner in his honor when he said, "If I knew I was going to live so long, I would have taken better care of myself." He wasn't kidding. And you shouldn't kid about your health, either.

One day of neck exercises won't do the trick for all time. The neck needs to be exercised regularly, as do all your other joints. So before you start today's shoulder limbering, go back and repeat yesterday's exercises for the neck. (Give yourself an extra Feeling Fine point for doing them.) Then resume reading.

Every joint has a natural physiological range of motion. When your neck is limber you'll be able to turn your head through almost 240 degrees. The elbow has about 150-degrees of motion. The arm can rotate from the shoulder through a full 360-degree turn. You need all 360 degrees to do even such simple things as picking things up off the floor or reaching above your head to screw in a light bulb.

If you play a sport that uses a racquet, club, or bat, you will particularly appreciate limber shoulders.

Here are some exercises to limber up those joints.

SHOULDER-SAVER ONE

1. Stand straight, with your arms at your sides.
2. Slowly swing your right arm in a full circle— as if you were doing the backstroke slowly. Be sure to do this in slow motion.

3. Repeat 10 times. Relax.

4. Do the same motions in the reverse direction 10 times.

5. Repeat both the forward and backward swings with your left arm 10 times each way.

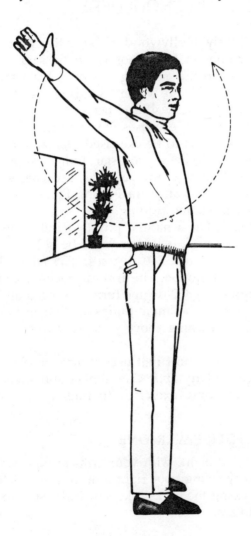

SHOULDER-SAVER TWO

1. Stand straight, with your arms at your sides.

2. Raise your right arm toward the ceiling, reaching as high as you can, as though changing a light bulb. Return your arm to your side.

3. Repeat 10 times.

4. Repeat the same motion with your left arm 10 times.

SHOULDER-SAVER THREE

1. Stand straight, with your arms at your sides.

2. Shrug your shoulders as high as your ears and rotate them forward, down, and then around to the back. This motion is similar to those you might make if an ice cube were dropped down your back or you had a back itch you couldn't quite reach.

3. Continue rolling your shoulders in a circle 10 times. Relax.

4. Repeat in the reverse direction 10 times.

Give yourself a Feeling Fine point for your neck limbering and another for your shoulders.

FEELING FINE POINTS
(Choose one or more from each category.)

GROWING PLEASURES
- [ ] **Balancing your goals**
- [ ] Spending $1 for fun
- [ ] Taking time alone

UNSTRESSING PLEASURES
- [ ] **Talking with your companion**
- [ ] Removing yourself from stress
- [ ] Paying attention to your target organs

EATING PLEASURES
- [ ] **Cutting back on sugar**
- [ ] Trimming back on fat
- [ ] Staying away from your target foods

BODY PLEASURES
- [ ] **Saving your shoulders**
- [ ] Giving your back some support
- [ ] Walking for pleasure

DAY 9

Growing Pleasures

GOALS: MAKING THINGS CLEAR

A goal reached is a joy.

A goal reached but unrecognized, a disappointment.

What good is a goal if you can't even tell when you've reached it? Not much good and not much fun. That's why it's essential to write clear, specific goals. All too often the goals we strive for are unrecognizable—even unreachable—because they don't have a clear end point, a moment when we know we have accomplished what we set out to do.

There's another advantage to having clearly defined goals. It's easier to know what must be done to achieve the goals. Let me give you an example of how making a fuzzy goal clearer also makes it easier to achieve.

Fuzzy Goal: "I want to be a better parent."

Now that's an admirable goal, but how will you know when you've achieved it? How will you even know if you're getting close? Will you ask your children? Your neighbors? How will you judge? What yardstick will you use? That goal is too general and it can't be measured. Because it can't be measured, you can't tell when it's been achieved. Let's state the same goal in a better way.

Clearer Goal: "I will be a better parent in the following ways:

    1. By spending ten minutes a day alone with each child.
    2. By reviewing homework with each child each night.
    3. By giving the children healthy snacks instead of candy.
    4. By saying at least one loving and encouraging thing to each child every day."

When restated in these clear and specific terms, the goal of becoming a better parent becomes an achievable task, and there's a recognizable end point at which it has, at least in part, been accomplished. It's clear what has to be done to achieve the goal, and it's easy to know whether one has reached it or not.

It should be easy to make clear goals in the financial category, but many people seem to have just as much trouble there. Let me give you another example:

Fuzzy Goal: "I'm going to put away some money to take care of the future."

That's a fine objective, too. Everyone should do it. But how will you know when the future is taken care of? How much is "some" money? What kind of future do you want? How much money will it take to insure it? You can't tell by looking at the goal. Here's a clearer way to write the same objective.

Clearer Goal: "Every month I'm going to put $150 into a savings account. To achieve this I will:

    1. Work four extra hours a week and put those earnings aside.
    2. Cut my expenses by $20 a week and put those savings into the bank."

Defining this financial objective more clearly won't make it fun to work longer and doesn't make it easy to cut costs. It will let you know exactly what needs to be done, and it will insure that you'll reach the goal as long as you follow the plan.

This technique makes sense not only for parental and financial goals but also for any kind of life goal. No good executive would try to manage a business without clear objectives. Why try to manage the business of your life without them? Let's put the technique to work for you today by making clear objectives out of the goals you've already written for yourself.

To earn your Feeling Fine point today, all you've got to do is review your goals, category by category, to see if they meet these criteria:

1. Are they clear?
2. Are they specific?
3. Are they measurable?
4. Will you know when you've reached them?

Review your own goals, make them specific, and give yourself a point for gaining control of your life.

Unstressing Pleasures

GUIDED IMAGERY AND PAIN RELIEF

Sometimes the best medicine isn't medicine.

For most people pain relief comes in the form of pills—500 million dollars' worth of pills every year in the United States. While those pills do remove some pain, they also leave many unpleasant side effects in place of the pain: ulcers, bleeding, nausea, rashes—the list is endless.

When pain is so severe that nothing else will work, pain pills may be worth the risk. But when the pain is caused by stress or tension, popping a pill isn't the answer. Then it's time to use the power of your thoughts to eliminate the discomfort from your body. Guided imagery can help you do it. Today we're going to show you a no-medicine (and no-side-effect) way to relieve pain. Let me tell you a story to show you one way guided imagery works.

Recently one of the neighborhood kids scared my ten-year-old son Steve out of his wits by sneaking up on him and letting out a blood-curdling yell. Steve flew into the house at ninety miles an hour. Five minutes later he was complaining of a stomachache.

I knew that stomachache was a direct result of the frightening experience, but I knew, too, that Steve would not accept that explanation, at least not from me. His pain seemed very real to him and he wanted some attention. Obviously I wasn't going to give him a pain pill. Instead I suggested that he lie down and use guided imagery to ask his creature-friend for advice. (Steve's creature is a fish named Flipper who is always willing to dispense advice which Steve is almost always willing to follow.) Fifteen minutes later Steve came back to me looking much better.

"What did Flipper tell you about your stomachache?" I asked.

"He said I got it because I was scared," Steve responded. "He told me to put a towel over the painful spot for five minutes. He said the pain would be gone when I took the towel off. He was right."

The towel wasn't curative. It merely allowed Steve to ease out of the pain gracefully. His awareness of the real cause of pain—the scare—allowed him to deal with the stress properly and eliminate the pain. Flipper was the tool that let my son be honest with himself.

We all have this inner diagnostician, a creature-adviser who can come to us in time of need. Our creatures may not have the proper degrees, but their brand of medicine works because they are not afraid to tell us when we're making ourselves sick. (Usually we're not afraid to hear it from our advisers, although it might make us angry if we heard the same thing from someone else, like a doctor.)

Using your creature is one way to use guided imagery to relieve pain. However, you don't always have to impose on your creature-friend to gain pain relief. There is another form of guided imagery which many of my patients have found helpful. They literally *visualize* their pain away.

Maybe you can do it, too? The next time you have a pain, give it a try. Find a place where you won't be disturbed. Make yourself comfortable in a chair, close your eyes, and try any or all of the following:

1. Visualize a light bulb and make it shine as brightly as you can. "Move" the light bulb to the area that is in pain—your elbow, your neck, your stomach, wherever. Pretend that the light is your pain. Then, very slowly turn the light down, as though you were turning a dimming switch, so that the light from the bulb gradually gets dimmer and dimmer. Take a few minutes to do this. As the light slowly fades, so should the pain.

2. Another way is to visualize a box. Imagine that you have put your pain into the box. Then for several minutes shrink the box smaller and smaller, until the box—and the pain inside it—are gone altogether.

3. If you prefer things nautical, put your pain in a boat. Send the boat away. As it slowly disappears over the horizon and out of view, so will your pain.

4. Imagine that your pain has a color (many people see it as an intense red). Slowly tone the color down. Go from bright red (or whatever color you choose) to light red to pink. Then start to imagine your pain as a "cooler" color, moving toward the green and blue side of the spectrum. The pain should "cool down," slowly fade away, and then disappear.

Do you have pain? Try guided imagery. You don't need a prescription and it doesn't cost a dime. And don't forget—your creature-friend doesn't play golf on Wednesdays and is always available for house calls.

Reach for guided imagery before you reach for a pill and you've earned another point for Feeling Fine.

Eating Pleasures

LIQUOR: HANDLE WITH CARE

Here's an easy one for you. What common item in the average American diet has none of the following nutrients?

Protein
Minerals
Vitamins A & D
B Vitamins
Vitamin C
Vitamin E

The answer is easy because the clue is in the title: alcoholic beverages. When it comes to nutrition, they have practically zero quality. No proteins, no vitamins, no minerals, no fiber. Only calories. At very high prices.

This kind of information would have helped my friend who complained, "I eat intelligently, but I can't keep my weight down."

True, he was a sensible eater. In a restaurant known for its exquisite man-sized steaks he had just ordered a green salad and charcoal-broiled spring chicken.

"You're eating right," I told him. "Your problem is the Old-Fashioned in your right hand."

"Wait," he protested, "I only have one of these a day. That's all."

Unfortunately, that's *not* all there is to it. Like most of us, my friend thinks about only one day at a time. He doesn't realize how many calories his drinks add up to over a year.

Let's figure it out.

His daily alcohol intake was approximately 180 calories. Not much if you think of it for only one day. But if he had stopped to figure it out, he would have seen that his moderate drinking comes to something like 65,000 calories in a year. That translates into roughly nineteen pounds!

Here are some other equivalents:

- One ounce of Scotch an evening—seventeen pounds a year.
- A three-ounce martini each night—eighteen pounds a year.
- Three nightly ounces of sherry—fifteen pounds a year.
- And beer—just two cans a night—will pack a whopping thirty-three pounds.

To understand the role liquor plays in your life, your task for today is to estimate the average number of drinks (wine, hard liquor, beer) you have each week and to multiply that figure by the approximate number of calories in each drink. Then multiply your weekly caloric intake—from alcohol alone—by fifty weeks (we'll give you two weeks off for good behavior) to come up with the total number of alcoholic calories you consume per year.

Here's another short list of the approximate calories in some alcoholic beverages to show you how this works:

• One four-ounce glass of red or white wine has 100 calories.

• One shot of Scotch, bourbon, vodka, gin, etc. has 70 calories (add 100 calories per drink if you use a mix).

• One twelve-ounce can of beer has 160 calories. So, if you have a mixed drink before dinner three times a week (170 calories × 3 days = 510 calories per week); a glass of wine with dinner every night (100 calories × 7 days = 700 calories per week); and an average of 3 cans of beer over the weekend (160 calories × 3 = 480 calories per week)—your weekly intake of alcohol amounts to 1,690 calories. Multiply the weekly total by fifty weeks to calculate your yearly intake of alcoholic calories.

Now, take that astronomical figure and divide it by 3,500—the number of calories in a pound of weight: _____. That's the number of pounds *your* liquor consumption puts on you in one year. Stop the liquor and that's the number of pounds you'll lose, unless you fill the void with something other than water, tea, or coffee.

Alcohol's weight-increasing effects don't stop with the drink itself. Liquor lowers our inhibitions and undermines our judgment, so we tend to eat peanuts, potato chips, crackers, and junk while we're drinking.

What are the alternatives?

If you are content with your weight and your drinking never interferes with your functioning, you probably don't need to worry about the alternatives. Studies have shown that people who drink very little do no worse than anyone else in terms of physical health and overall survival. You might want to consider, however, that you could be providing yourself with more interesting foods in place of alcohol.

If you'd like to lose weight you ought to cut down on alcoholic beverages. Just don't substitute anything high-calorie in their place.

Here are a few ways to help keep the alcohol calories down when you *do* drink:

1. Stick with lower-proof drinks. The higher the proof of the alcohol, the greater its caloric content. For example, one and a half ounces of 80-proof liquor has 95 calories, but the same amount of 90-proof has 110 calories.

2. Order drinks straight. Regular mixes (especially those used in restaurants and bars) add about 100 calories to your drink.

3. In mixed drinks ask for half a shot instead of the usual full one.

4. Make your drinks tall by filling the glass with ice. Dilute the alcohol and fill yourself up with water.

5. If you like a mix, switch to soda.

6. Avoid exotic drinks. Irish coffee has almost 175 calories, a daiquiri 177 calories, a zombie more than 500.

7. If you drink wine, choose a dry wine. It has fewer calories than a sweet one.

8. Limit yourself to one drink.

And here are some ways to avoid the fattening munchies that come with the drinks:

• In a bar ask the waiter or waitress to remove peanuts and chips from the table.

• At home serve fresh-cut vegetables as appetizers. Carrot and celery sticks, cauliflower, slices of cucumber and zucchini are the greatest.

• Serve low-calorie dips. Substitute cottage cheese for sour cream in the recipe and you'll cut the calories in half.

Give yourself one Feeling Fine point whenever you incorporate one of these suggestions into your day.

Body Pleasures

LIMBERING UP TO SAVE YOUR HIPS AND KNEES

Today we're at the joints that help put a lot of zest into your life—the hips and knees. Walking, climbing stairs, dancing, bicycling—where would you be without a good pair of hips and knees? Today these are what we're going to limber up.

First do some neck limbering. Give yourself a point when you do. Then limber your shoulders. Give yourself another point.

Now let's get to the hips and knees.

KNEE-SAVER ONE

1. Lie on your back on the floor, with your legs straight.

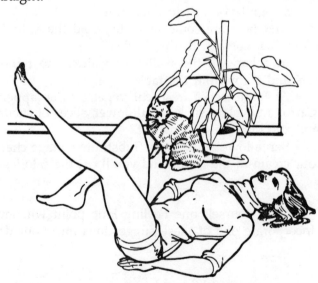

2. Put your hands, palms down, under your buttocks.

3. Lift both legs up, knees bent, and pretend you are riding a bicycle. Make *slow* pedaling motions for 15 rounds.

KNEE-SAVER TWO

1. Stand with both feet together.

2. Raise your right knee and grasp it with both hands.

3. Pull it straight up—slowly—toward your chest, keeping your back straight.

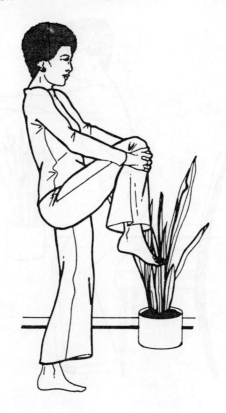

4. Lower your leg to floor.

5. Repeat 10 times.

6. Do the same with the left leg 10 times. (This one is great for the hips, too.)

KNEE-SAVER THREE

1. Stand in front of a chair with your back toward it.

2. Hold your arms out in front of you for balance, bend your knees, and pretend you are going to sit down.

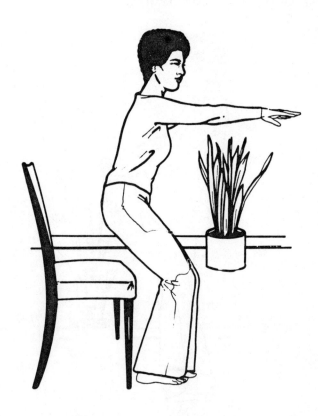

3. Get your bottom as close to the chair as you can, but don't sit.

4. Straighten up and return to the standing position.

5. Repeat 10 times.

HIP-SAVER ONE

1. While standing on your left leg, bend your right knee and grasp the outside of your ankle with both hands.

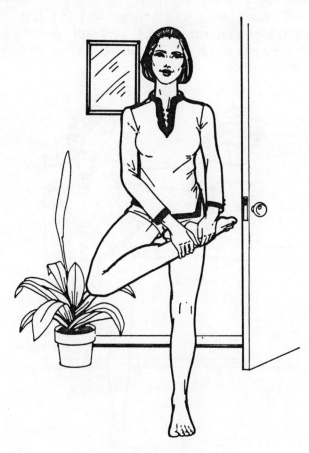

2. Trying to keep your body straight, slowly lift your ankle upward and to the left, attempting to touch your left hip with your right heel. If you can do this easily, you're limber enough. If you can't reach the hip, don't worry—with practice you should soon be able to.

3. Repeat the process 5 times with each leg.

HIP-SAVER TWO

1. Stand with your arms stretched straight out to the sides and your feet together.

2. Keep your toes pointed forward and raise your right leg to the side as high as it will go—trying to touch your right hand. Don't bend your knee. Return to beginning position.

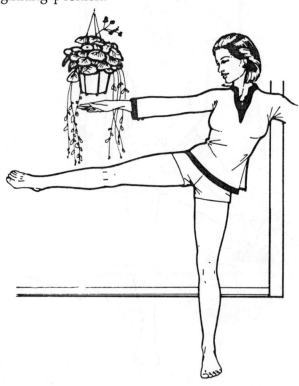

3. Slowly raise the leg forward as high as you can. Return to the standing position.

4. Slowly raise the leg backward as far as you can without falling over. Do the sequence 5 times.

5. Repeat with the left leg 5 times.

Give yourself a Feeling Fine point for every joint you limbered.

FEELING FINE POINTS
(Choose one or more from each category.)

GROWING PLEASURES

☐ **Sharpening your goals**

☐ Finding new goals to sharpen

☐ Saying I love you/I like you

UNSTRESSING PLEASURES

☐ **Relieving pain through guided imagery**

☐ Easing stress with guided imagery

☐ Removing a cause of stress from your environment

EATING PLEASURES

☐ **Being careful with liquor**

☐ Putting fiber in your diet

☐ Skipping calories

BODY PLEASURES

☐ **Saving your hips and knees**

☐ Breathing deeply

☐ Enjoying self-massage

DAY 10

Growing Pleasures

GOALS: FACING REALITY

Few things in life are more frustrating than working toward a goal and failing, only to realize later that for reasons you never thought about, the mission was almost impossible from the start. Or perhaps the goal was not worth the price you had to pay to accomplish it.

Clearly it's foolish to set your heart on becoming Chairman of the Board when the position is already filled by the person who owns all the company's stock (and who's only 35). It's a sure source of frustration to try to be the neatest housekeeper in the land when you're also working full-time and trying to bring up three kids. You've little chance of success if your goal is to be the tennis champion at the park when you've only got time to play twice a week.

I'm not suggesting that you avoid all difficult goals. Overcoming an appropriate amount of challenge is necessary for any real satisfaction. What I am saying is that to achieve your goals they have to be something you can reasonably expect to accomplish, given the obstacles in your path. They must be realistic.

How can you determine if your goals are realistic? By taking into account the things most likely to keep you from achieving them. And those limitations aren't always as obvious as in the examples above.

Everybody has limitations. Limitations imposed

by the time available to us, by our finances, by our natural talents, and by our responsibilities to the important people in our lives. If you don't give consideration to the limitations in your life, you might end up choosing unrealistic and unrealizable goals. Today look at the goals you've been putting together for the past three days and ask yourself the following questions:

1. *How realistic are your goals in terms of your time schedule?* Everything takes a little longer than you think. If you give yourself the extra time before you start, you won't spoil the fun of achieving the goal because you couldn't get it done in time. Setting goals that are time-realistic means fewer frustrations, less pressure, and more fun along the way. Setting a realistic time schedule will also help you decide if a goal is really worth the time investment you have to make to obtain it.

Don't set up all your goals so that you have to accomplish them simultaneously. If you have some that you can do immediately, others that will take a few months, and a few that may even take years, your chances of reaching them—on time—will be much greater.

2. *How realistic are your goals financially?* Most of us have a pretty fair idea of whether we have the money to do the things and buy the goods we want. But that's not the only way to determine whether you can afford your goals financially. You should also consider what the cost of earning the dollars will be to your health, and the cost of spending them to your peace of mind. Taking an affordable vacation somewhere nearby will leave you feeling a lot more relaxed than spending a week at a jet-set resort and then returning home tense with worry about how you're going to pay the bill. Sometimes when you fly now and pay later, the cost has to be figured in more than money.

3. *Are your goals realistic for your natural abilities?* It's great to have goals that challenge you to do better or

to be better. But goals that are out of harmony with your natural abilities are apt to lead to frustration as you try to achieve them. Why try to become a singer when you can't carry a tune? Why study accounting when numbers aren't your game? You don't have to give up music. Learn to play the guitar. You don't have to give up business. You've just got to find your strengths.

The fact is, we don't all have the same natural equipment. Goals that are based on exploiting your strengths are the ones you are most likely to accomplish.

4. *Are your goals realistic in terms of opposition from others?* Many times worthwhile goals may be thwarted because someone else (a husband, a wife, a boss) doesn't want you to reach them. Sometimes their reasons are good, sometimes not. But whatever the reason it's important to realize that not everyone wants you to get where you'd like to go. You have to take other people's objections into consideration when you set goals. Don't give up important ones because of some interference, but don't waste time on goals that may well be impossible to attain over the objections and obstacles imposed by others.

Think realistically about your goals and give yourself a Feeling Fine point.

Unstressing Pleasures

PREPARING FOR SLEEP

What is a "good" night's sleep? Above all, it means you get up feeling refreshed. Researchers have found that a good night's sleep is fairly complicated. It consists of repeated cycles during which we go from a light sleep to a deep sleep and back to light sleep again. Each cycle lasts about ninety minutes and consists of several stages.

During stages 1 and 2 slumber is very light—so light, in fact, that people who spend the whole night in these stages usually get up the next morning and say, "I didn't sleep a wink all night." People who feel the most rested after a night's sleep are the ones who get down to stages 3 and 4—the deepest stages—during most of their ninety-minute sleep cycles.

Sleep is essential for good health. The body uses this time to rebalance certain physiologic processes, although researchers still cannot tell us how the body does it. One thing they have discovered: not everyone needs the same amount of sleep to avoid body fatigue. There are some people who actually get only three or four hours of sleep per night and thrive! Others can't make it through the day if they don't get nine or ten. Most of us need seven or eight hours of *good* sleep. When we don't get it we suffer (often the world around us suffers, too).

The older we get the less sleep we need. Babies need almost eighteen hours a day, adolescents about eight to ten, and most senior citizens need less than they did during their middle years. (Many older people think they have insomnia because they can't stay asleep as long as they used to, but they don't realize that needing less sleep is normal.)

If you ever have trouble getting a good night's sleep, I've got some help for you. You don't need to be a chronic insomniac to need help—everyone has a poor night once in a while. Here are nine tips to use for getting to sleep more quickly, sleeping more deeply, and waking up more refreshed.

1. Cooperate with your ninety-minute sleep cycles. Don't go to bed unless you are sleepy, no matter

what the clock says. And when you do get sleepy, don't put off going to bed.

2. Avoid such stimulants as coffee, tea, and cola drinks before bedtime. Instead try a glass of warm milk, hot chocolate, or soup.

3. If you smoke, avoid smoking before bedtime. For some, nicotine is as strong a stimulant as coffee. If you must put something in your mouth, try an apple.

4. If you exercise vigorously, do it early in the day. That will help you sleep better at night. Don't exercise too close to bedtime. That will mobilize your muscles and stimulate your mind—not the best state to be in for sleep. If you want to do exercises late in the day, do isometrics or stretching exercises. They're okay because the stretching and contraction causes muscles to relax totally afterward—just the thing for sound sleeping. More about this tomorrow.

5. Avoid late-night TV chillers and action-packed books. If you begin *The Day of the Jackal* just before bedtime, as I once did, you may not be able to put it down until you finish. (When I finished, I *really* couldn't sleep.)

6. Use a clock-radio that shuts itself off after thirty minutes. Play relaxing music to put yourself to sleep.

7. Don't nap during the day. If you feel fatigued try guided imagery or go for a brisk ten-minute walk, but don't nap. (I once had a friend who went to the beach for a week's vacation, dozed on the sand, took a nap before dinner, and then wondered why he had trouble sleeping.)

8. If you want to eat before bedtime, make it a small snack. Your stomach doesn't stop digesting just because you've gone to bed, and a big meal will keep you awake.

9. Go to bed with a cheerful thought.

Use these tips to get a good night's sleep and give yourself a point for Feeling Fine in the morning.

Eating Pleasures

VITAMINS: THE ABC'S OF GOOD HEALTH

I wish I had never heard the word.
I wish they weren't so important.
I wish I could ignore them.

But I *have* heard the word, and vitamins *are* essential, so I won't ignore them. I'll tell you what I think about them, even though I know the mail will start pouring in, as it did when I talked about vitamins on television. It seemed that the whole country was divided into two groups: those who disagreed with me because I recommended too many vitamins and those who disagreed with me because I recommended too few. Why is it that people who agree with me don't write letters?

To make it easy for myself later on I've decided to answer all the questions now. Here goes:

Question: Are vitamins essential for good health?

Answer: Yes. Absolutely yes.

Question: Can the average American get enough vitamins from the food he or she eats?

Answer: There's nothing wrong with the "average American." It's the "average American diet" that's so bad. Almost all of us can get enough vitamins from our normal diet if we're willing to work at it. The trouble is, many people aren't willing to spend the time, thought, and money it takes to eat well. Some people have special problems preparing a truly nutritious diet. For example: poor people (who can't afford to buy all the foods they need); old people (whose bodies don't absorb nutrients well); single people (who find it hard to prepare a balanced diet without wasting a lot of food); frequent travelers (who never know what kind of food they're getting or how it has been prepared); dieters (who may not be taking in enough food to meet the minimum nutritional needs).

Question: What should people who can't get enough vitamins in their diet do?

Answer: Take multiple-vitamin supplements. But they should never forget that a poor diet plus vitamins is still a poor diet.

Question: Which vitamins and how much should we take?

Answer: Vitamins A and D: *never* more than the Recommended Daily Allowance (RDA) established by the National Research Council. Vitamin C: about three times the RDA. All others: the RDA is probably all that's needed.

Question: Don't vitamins always make you feel better?

Answer: Absolutely not. Some people report they feel worse when they take vitamins. Many people say Vitamin E makes them sick, and others break out in a rash every time they take Vitamin C. Very high doses of both of those vitamins have been associated with significant side effects in *some* people. Remember that not everyone reacts the same way to anything; why should vitamins be any exception? Also remember that high doses of Vitamins A and D have been *proved dangerous* to almost everyone. Never exceed the RDA with these two vitamins.

Question: Is there a difference between natural and synthetic vitamins?

Answer: Natural vitamins cost more. People are more likely to have allergic reactions to the natural vitamins, because there is a higher potential for them to be contaminated with other materials. People who are allergic to wheat germ are more likely to react

badly to "Natural E" than the synthetic form. Otherwise, the biologic effects are the same, whether
natural or synthetic.

Question: Do some people need more vitamins than
others?

Answer: Yes. Among those who do are the following
groups: smokers; women using birth control pills;
the chronically ill; people taking anti-tuberculous
medications; people under great stress; alcoholics.
Almost all people in these groups should be taking a
multi-vitamin supplement.

Question: How do I earn my Feeling Fine point today?

Answer: Eat a healthy diet and promise you won't write
to me about vitamins.

Body
Pleasures

LIMBERING UP TO
SAVE YOUR BACK

"Oh, my aching back!"

That expression is no joke for the millions who
suffer from chronic low-back pain. Unlike acute back
strain, where proper treatment and a few days' rest in
bed make you as good as new, chronic low-back pain just
seems to go on forever.

Usually the best way to treat a chronic backache
is with exercise. That's also the best way to prevent it. So
you don't have to have a bad back to be interested in
today's limbering.

There are some very simple principles to follow.
If you have a weak area in your back, you need to
strengthen it. If you have a tight area, you need to loosen

it. And you must exercise every day, whether it hurts or not. That's a small price to pay for freedom from chronic, nagging pain.

Here are some exercises to help keep your back healthy.

BACK-SAVER ONE

1. Lie on your back with your arms stretched out to the sides.

2. Lift your right leg and swing it gently toward your left hand, keeping your leg as straight as possible. Don't "throw" the leg—just lift it up and over, slowly and gently. Try to keep both shoulders on the floor.

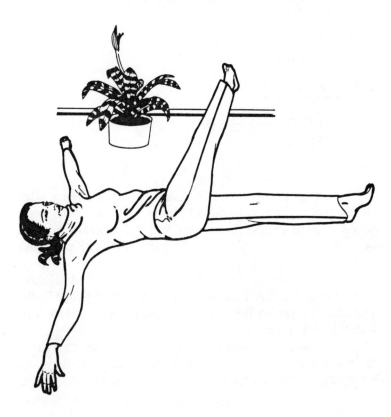

3. Return your leg slowly to the original position.

4. Repeat 10 times.

5. Repeat process with the left leg 10 times.

BACK-SAVER TWO

1. Lie on your back with your knees bent, feet flat on the floor, and arms stretched out to the sides.

2. Flatten the small of your back against the floor. Tighten your abdominal muscles as well as your buttocks.

3. Hold for a count of 5, then relax. Don't hold your breath; just breathe normally.

4. Repeat 10 times.

BACK-SAVER THREE

1. Lie on your back with your knees bent and feet flat on the floor.

2. Clasp your right knee with both hands and slowly bring the knee up to your chest.

3. Hold for a count of 10, then return leg to the floor.

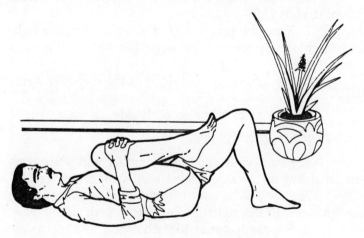

4. Repeat 5 times.

5. Repeat process with left knee 5 times.

6. Then clasp both knees and bring them to your chest simultaneously.

7. Hold for a count of 10, then lower the legs to the starting position.

8. Repeat 5 times.

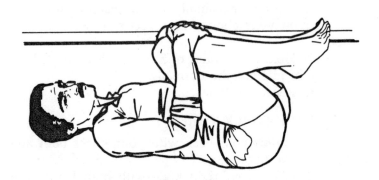

BACK-SAVER FOUR

1. Stand with your feet together and your arms down at your sides.

2. Bend the upper part of your body to the right and reach slowly toward the floor. Go only as far as is comfortable.

3. Straighten up and do it in the opposite direction.

4. Repeat 10 times to each side.

BACK-SAVER FIVE

1. Stand with your feet together and your arms stretched out to the sides, level with your shoulders.

2. *Slowly* twist your trunk to the left as far as you can go, then to the right. Never throw your arms!

3. Repeat 10 times to each side.

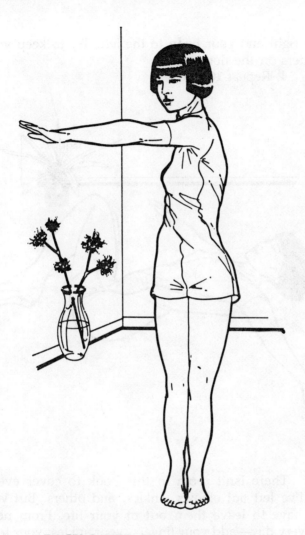

BACK-SAVER SIX

1. Lie on your back with your arms stretched out to the sides.

2. Draw your knees up to your chest.

3. Slowly roll your legs and thighs to the left and the upper part of your body to the right, then roll the legs

to the right and your body to the left. Try to keep your shoulders on the floor.

    4. Repeat 10 times.

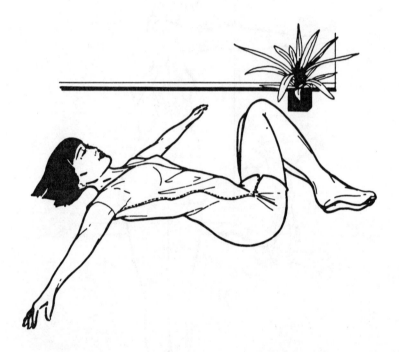

There isn't room in this book to cover every joint. I've left out elbows, ankles, and others. But you don't have to leave them out of your life. From now on—every day—add your fingers, your ankles, your toes to the routine. Move each one as far as it will go several times a day, and you'll be able to enjoy free movement for years.

Give yourself a Feeling Fine point for building a better back.

FEELING FINE POINTS
(Choose one or more from each category.)

GROWING PLEASURES
☐ **Checking your goals for realism**
☐ Spending $1 for fun
☐ Appreciating someone
   UNSTRESSING PLEASURES
☐ **Getting a good night's sleep**
☐ Talking with your guided-imagery companion
☐ Removing yourself from stressful environments
   EATING PLEASURES
☐ **Paying heed to vitamins**
☐ Cutting sugar
☐ Substituting few calories for many
   BODY PLEASURES
☐ **Saving your back**
☐ Limbering the rest of you
☐ Breathing deeply

DAY 11

Growing Pleasures

GOALS: GOING AFTER WHAT YOU WANT

During the several days you've been looking at your goals you've had a chance to define them, balance them, clarify them, and modify them. Now it's time to start achieving them. Today all you need to do to earn a Feeling Fine point is take the first step toward achieving one goal in each goal category.

It's easy to take the first step when goals are short term, simple, and clear-cut. In some instances taking the first step may also mean you've taken the final step. That's true if the goal is something like cleaning up the house. Sometimes the first step puts you on a direct path toward the final goal, like opening a savings account when you need to save enough money for a vacation or a new car.

Getting started on most goals, however, requires a different kind of first step: planning. Carefully laying out the steps to accomplish your long-range goals is a vital part of accomplishing them.

The best way to do your planning is on paper. Writing down plans for the future changes them from dreams into objectives. It makes them more concrete and enhances your commitment to them. Writing down the individual steps makes the goals easier to achieve.

Planning on paper will be a lot easier if you follow some simple rules.

1. *Break it up.* The most difficult tasks become

simpler when you divide them into sequential steps. Break down into the smallest possible parts what needs to be done to reach your goal. Then instead of a complex job that may look like more than you can possibly handle, all you'll be facing is a series of achievable steps. Attaining your goal will become a matter of doing one small thing at a time.

2. *Make measurable milestones.* Do you remember how satisfying it was to pass the mileage markers on your last auto trip and know each time that you were getting closer and closer to your destination? The same thing is true when you're traveling toward a goal in life: good markers allow you to measure your progress and tell you when you've strayed from the most direct pathway to your goal. Make the markers clear and look for them frequently.

Remember also that you can't always maintain the same speed on the road, so don't expect steady and uninterrupted movement toward your goal. And don't get impatient. That's the best way to take a wrong turn.

3. *Reward yourself along the way.* As you conquer short-term goals and move closer to the more distant or complicated objectives, don't forget to reward yourself. Sometimes committing yourself to a goal in one area means depriving yourself in another. Don't let it turn into total deprivation. That's not what achieving goals is all about. Reward yourself for a job half done and then again, when you've finished.

4. *Review your list periodically.* Just because you had a goal once doesn't mean you have to have it forever. Every six months go back over your list and revise it. If something on the list no longer seems worth doing, take that goal off your list. Replace it with a new one that has more meaning and reward in it.

Get moving toward your goals now and give yourself another Feeling Fine point.

Unstressing Pleasures

WHEN YOU HAVE TROUBLE SLEEPING

Sleep is one of the best de-stressing techniques nature has given us. But if you have trouble sleeping you are not alone. One out of every three people say they have some sort of problem with their sleep. The trouble is, many people who have trouble sleeping rely on a solution that only makes matters worse: they cover up their sleeping problem with a sleeping pill.

Sleeping pills do indeed put you to sleep, but you don't sleep well. People who use pills to sleep don't spend enough time in the deep stages of sleep and don't dream as much as normal, both of which are essential for health. People who use sleeping pills regularly can become depressed and irritable, have trouble concentrating, lose coordination, and suffer blurred vision. Even an occasional sleeping pill can leave a hangover the next morning.

Regular sleeping-pill users also develop tolerance—they require larger and larger doses of medicine just to achieve the same effect. And if they try to stop the pills they get a dream "rebound"—they have nightmares. Then a vicious circle begins. They have to take even higher doses of drugs just to keep the nightmares from occurring. The pills become the problem instead of the solution.

For some sleep problems there are simple solutions. Others were not made in a day and will not go away in a day. Take a look at this list and see which of the sleep problems and the recommended solutions fit you.

Unfinished Business. If this is your problem, don't take it to bed with you. Did you forget to pay the bills? Get out of bed and write the checks. Do you have to prepare a proposal for the boss? Got a term paper due? Get out of bed and do the work! Don't let unfinished business keep your mind busy and keep you awake.

Anticipation. If you are thinking about things you need to do tomorrow and you can't sleep because of it, get up and write them down. Put them down on paper and you can get them off your mind. Don't return to bed until you're sure there's nothing left to think about.

Unresolved Conflicts. Fight with your wife? Compromise before you turn in. Disagreement with a friend? Get on the phone and talk it out. If it's too late, write it out. Writing it down lets you get the feelings off your mind. It will also serve as a rehearsal for a face-to-face talk in the morning.

Aches and Pains. You've done it again. Gone skiing without getting in shape first. Played football with the neighborhood kids. Dusted off your bike and rode ten miles. And you ache all over. You vow you won't do it again, but that doesn't help you now. The solution: try a long, hot shower or tub bath. Use a hot-water bottle. If nothing else works, take some aspirin or acetaminophen (an over-the-counter aspirin substitute) to dull the ache. Try using guided imagery for pain relief, too.

Situational Problems. Some problem got you down? Get out of bed! Spend half an hour thinking about it. Make some notes on how to deal with it. Then go back to bed. Make your bed a place to sleep, not worry. If you make a habit of worrying in bed you'll find that just getting into bed will be a cue to start worrying.

Depression. This is one of the most common causes of sleeping problems and one of the hardest to treat. When you're really down, no simple little trick is going to make you sleep perfectly (although some of the techniques described here and others I'll show you later may help greatly). You've got to get to the basic problem and work on that. You don't have to solve it completely. Just make a little progress in the right direction and watch your sleep improve dramatically.

Obviously I can do no more about depression in this book than encourage you to reach out for help. Ask friends, counselors, or your doctor for advice. When their advice fits you, try it. You'll be surprised how much better that can make you feel—and sleep.

Give yourself a Feeling Fine point for using these tips to get a better night's sleep.

Eating
Pleasures

ADDITIVES: NOT QUITE FRESH-OFF-THE-FARM

Question: If food manufacturers decided to cancel all the additives mixed into their products at the rate of one a day, how long would it take before all products were free of additives?

Answer: About fourteen years—because an estimated 5,000 additives are in use.

Some additives are natural foods themselves, used to enhance flavor or to keep food from spoiling—like salt, which is one of the oldest and best preservatives known. Citric acid is another example of a preservative which is really a food itself. It appears naturally in oranges and lemons and is added to beef and pork cuts to maintain them during storage. Calcium propionate is another—it appears naturally in Swiss cheese and is used artificially to preserve bread.

In some cases it may be safer to eat foods with additives than without them. An example of this is unsaturated vegetable oil. When it is exposed to the air for even a very short time it oxidizes and forms chemical compounds called peroxides, which some scientists believe cause cancer. Chemical preservatives like BHT and BHA are added to vegetable oil to keep it from oxidizing and going rancid. Anything made with vegetable oil (like crackers) also needs something like BHT. Many nutritionists now believe that given a choice between eating spoiled vegetable oil or BHT, you're probably a lot safer with the additive.

But some additives are used only to "pretty up" a food—to change its color or improve its consistency. It's hard to justify their use in many cases. Why do we have to have bright green pears or bright red cherries? Why can't we learn to live with their natural colors?

It seems that every time we open the newspaper we read about another food dye or additive on the suspect list. Cyclamates and cancer. Red dye and cancer. Food dyes and hyperactive kids. Now it's saccharin and cancer.

What should you do? The answer is fairly simple. Don't eat additives when you can avoid them. Here are some things you can do to cut down the amount of additives you get.

1. *Never* buy food with coloring added if you've got another choice.

2. If you have time, shop more frequently and stick to fresh or frozen meats and vegetables rather than canned.

3. Avoid processed meats—dried or canned luncheon meats, bacon, sausages, etc.

4. Cut down your intake of foods, such as hot dogs, which contain nitrites and nitrates.

5. Bake your own bread and pastries without preservatives, or buy those that do not have preservatives added. Store them in the freezer or refrigerator, or they will spoil.

6. Grow your own vegetables. A large percentage of the households in America now do.

7. Avoid chemical enhancers like MSG (monosodium glutamate). Some people get severe headaches, faintness, or numbness if they eat foods containing this ingredient. Since MSG is used a lot in Oriental cooking, its bad effects have been called the "Chinese Syndrome" by doctors.

8. Read the nutrition labels on foods and look for the products which contain little or no chemical additives. They're not hard to find—if you look for them.

If you buy foods without preservatives, you'll have to handle them more carefully in your own home; otherwise, you'll be throwing out a lot of spoiled food. Don't leave leftovers out after a meal; this gives bacteria a chance to grow. Place them in tightly covered containers and put them in the refrigerator or freezer right away.

Before eating food that has been stored for awhile, check for spoilage. If it has mold or a bad odor, don't eat it.

Today's point-getting activity requires little more than reaching and reading. Pick at least ten items off the shelves of your cupboards and refrigerator and read the labels. See how many of them contain additives or dyes that you could avoid if you shopped differently. Then give yourself a Feeling Fine point for not adding additives.

Body
Pleasures

STRETCHING: THE SHORT
AND LONG OF IT

What good is a big muscle if it hurts every time you move it? What good are beautiful biceps if you can't straighten your arms out all the way? For years the measure of a good muscle was how much weight it could lift. That *is* what counts if you're a professional weight lifter or a piano mover. But if you're an average person, it's not more strength you need, it's flexibility and freedom from pain. That's what stretching is all about.

Dancers have been doing stretching exercises for years. Now stretching techniques are being further developed to prevent many of the injuries experienced by competitive athletes. You never saw better calves and thighs than on those muscle-bound gridiron heroes. Trouble is, every Saturday and Sunday they had to carry dozens of them off the field on stretchers. Every TV commentator knew what to call those injuries. You heard terms like "hamstring muscle pull" and "collateral ligament strain" and "Achilles tendon tear." Those muscles and ligaments and tendons were pulling and straining and tearing right in front of your eyes.

The experts studied the problem and found the cause. Even in those well-trained athletes, muscles and connective tissues could not stand the stress of a *sudden* stretch. The solution? Pre-game stretching. The result? A dramatic decrease in injuries. There isn't a pro coach now who'd let his team start a game without stretching— *gradually*—beforehand. What is important to those beautiful physical specimens should become important to you.

During the next three days we'll give you an introduction to some basic stretching exercises. If you do these together with your limbering activities, you'll find yourself able to move extra inches in all directions. More important, you'll be able to do it without pain or injury. Before we start let's examine a few general principles about stretching.

There are two parts to "the stretch." In the first part you are merely extending yourself to the natural limit of your body's movement *at that time*. It's a limit which stretching exercises can extend greatly.

The second part of the stretch is called the developmental part. In this phase, you move just a little beyond your old natural limit until you reach a point where you can *feel* the stretch. You shouldn't feel pain, but you will feel your tissues pulling back against you. This is the position which will give you increased flexibility and new limits. This is a position of growth.

The difference between your first and final positions may be no more than ⅛ to ¼ inch, but there may be a great difference in the way they feel to you. Neither position should ever feel painful. If it does, you're stretching too far. As you move along you will be starting most sessions at a point more flexible than the initial position of your prior session. Before you start, here are some tips to make stretching work better for you:

1. Always do your stretching slowly and steadily. Rapid, jerky motions are the best way to stretch too far. As you do your stretching exercises, you will simply stretch until you feel your tissues pulling against you. That's the position you hold. If those tissues *hurt*, that's your signal to back off.

2. Don't stretch while "cold." Warm your body up with some limbering, and loosen yourself up with some shaking before you stretch yourself to your limit.

3. When you're stretching one part of your body,

try to keep all the other parts relaxed. Breathe naturally. Concentrate on nothing but the part being stretched.

    4. Don't try to do it all in a day. Only stretch the recommended number of times at the beginning. Don't hold a stretch longer than the recommended time at first. Later on when you become more flexible, you can begin to "stretch it out" if it feels good to you.

    Right now let's get started. If you haven't done so already, limber up and shake out so you'll be ready to stretch.

TOTAL BODY STRETCHER ONE

    1. Lie on your back with your arms extended over your head and your legs stretched straight out.

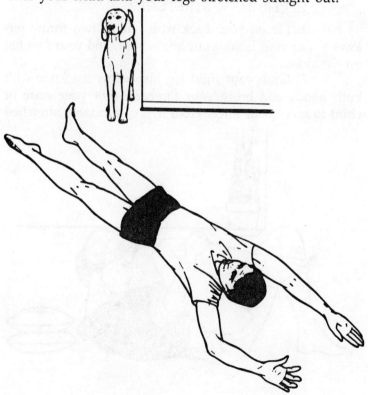

2. Point your toes, extend your fingers, and reach out as far as you can with your hands and feet. Hold the stretch for 5 to 10 seconds. Relax.

3. Repeat 3 times.

TOTAL BODY STRETCHER TWO

1. Lie on your back with your arms extended over your head and your legs stretched straight out.

2. Relax your right leg and left arm, and stretch your right arm and left leg (toes pointed) simultaneously. Then reverse sides. Hold each stretch for 5 to 10 seconds. Relax.

3. Repeat the process 3 times.

UPPER-BACK STRETCHER

1. Lie on your back with one or two throw pillows under your head, your knees bent, and your feet flat on the floor.

2. Grab your right leg just below the knee with both hands and bring your forehead (not your nose or chin) to meet your knee. Hold in a comfortably stretched

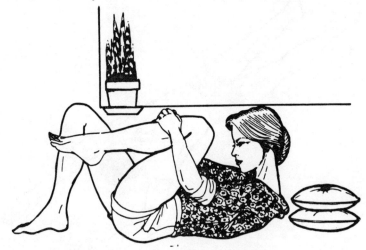

position for 5 to 10 seconds. If you can't touch your forehead to your knee at first, don't be distressed. Soon you'll be doing it easily.

3. Repeat 3 times.

4. Repeat process with left leg 3 times.

LOWER-BACK STRETCHER

1. Lie on your back with one or two throw pillows under your head, your knees bent, and your feet flat on the floor.

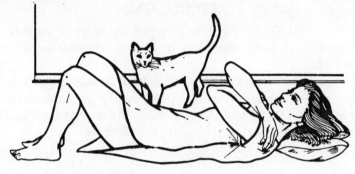

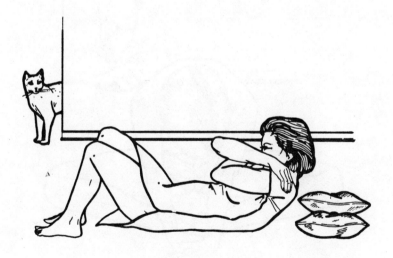

2. Cross your arms over your chest so that your right hand is on your left shoulder and your left hand on your right shoulder.

3. Sit up slowly, lifting your shoulder blades off the floor and trying to touch your forehead to your knees. Keep your chin on your chest as you sit up. Push up that little bit extra until you get the stretched feeling.

4. Start with 3 repetitions and build up a little each day until you can do it 10 times.

GROIN STRETCHER ONE

1. Sit on the floor and put the soles of your feet together, pulling your heels in as close to your crotch as possible.

2. Grasp your toes with both hands. Gently pull your head toward your feet until you feel a good stretch on the insides of your thighs. Hold the stretch for 5 to 10 seconds. You may also feel it in your back.

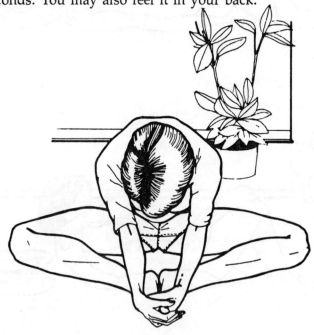

GROIN STRETCHER TWO

1. Assume the original position in Groin Stretcher One.

2. This time place your hands under your ankles with your forearms resting on the sides of your calves.

3. Gently press your forearms against your legs, trying to touch your knees to the floor. Hold the position for 5 to 10 seconds. You'll feel the stretch along the insides of your thighs.

4. Start with 3 repetitions and build up to 10. Over time, as you repeat this stretching exercise you will be able to bring your heels in closer and closer to the groin and your legs will lie flatter on the floor.

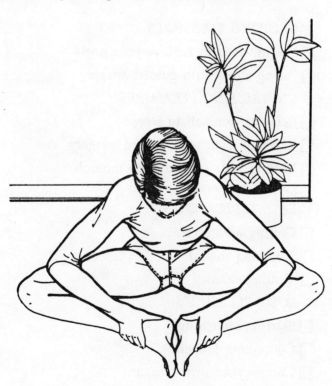

STANDING BODY STRETCHER

1. Stand with your feet about 6 inches apart.
2. Interlock your fingers and raise your arms over your head.
3. Stretch your arms up toward the ceiling as far as you can reach. Hold for about 15 seconds. Relax.
4. Repeat 10 times.

For limbering first, give yourself a Feeling Fine point. Stretch it to two for stretching.

FEELING FINE POINTS
(Choose one or more from each category.)

GROWING PLEASURES

☐ **Taking steps to achieve your goals**

☐ Easing stress with guided imagery

UNSTRESSING PLEASURES

☐ **Relaxing yourself to sleep**

☐ Relieving pain with guided imagery

☐ Visiting your private place through guided imagery

EATING PLEASURES

☐ **Cutting additives**

☐ Trimming the fat

☐ Cutting calories

BODY PLEASURES

☐ **Starting stretching**

☐ Continuing limbering

☐ Choose your own pleasure

DAY 12

Growing Pleasures

SLEEPING ON IT

One night a German chemist named Kekulé von Stradonitz had a dream in which he saw a snake biting its own tail. He awakened realizing that—in his sleep—he had visualized the solution to a complex scientific problem he had been struggling with.

Perhaps you've had a similar experience. You went to bed mulling over a problem or puzzle, had a dream about it, and woke up feeling inspired with a solution. If this happened to you, you may have written it off as a fluke. Don't dismiss your dreams so lightly. Think of them, instead, as messages to yourself.

On the average you dream three times a night —more than a thousand times a year. Some dreams are bizarre, some pedestrian, some amusing. One or two might be terrifying enough to bring you to a heart-thumping awakening. Whatever they are, those dreams are messages from parts of your mind with which you aren't in conscious touch. Those messages can tell you things about yourself that can be used to help you feel fine during your waking hours.

Many people say they cannot remember dreams in the morning, or that they can remember them only for a minute after they wake up. If that's your problem, here are some tips to help you to remember those dreams.

1. *Program yourself.* Before you go to sleep tonight (and from now on) tell yourself that on waking up in the morning you will remember all your dreams.

2. *Keep paper and pencil next to your bed.* As soon as you wake up, write down everything you can remember. Pretend the dream is still going on and you'll be more likely to recall much of it.

3. *Set your alarm ten minutes earlier than usual.* You may wake up in the middle of a dream, because the last dream each night usually occurs just before your normal waking hour.

Now, what do you do with this dream matter? Have fun with it. Learn from it. Look over your notes and see if you can come up with an interpretation. (The creature-adviser you found during guided imagery may have some ideas.) At first your dreams may be confusing and appear not to make any sense, but if you work with them awhile, you may begin to discover some valuable meanings.

When you look for meaning in your dreams, your first interpretation could be fairly literal. If you dreamed you were hurt in a skidding car, maybe you were reminding yourself to buy some new tires.

If you dreamed you were being beaten up in a fight, maybe you were revealing to yourself how you really feel about some situation in your waking life.

But if that kind of interpretation doesn't produce results, try looking for a more symbolic meaning. In case you have no idea where to start, here are a few common dream themes and some of their possible meanings.

• A dream that you have missed a bus, plane, or train may mean that you are afraid that life is passing you by—that you are "missing the boat" and will never fulfill your personal or career ambitions.

• A dream that a telephone number you dial is constantly busy, that the phone rings but no one answers, that you knock at doors that don't open, may be telling you that you are worrying about getting through to someone, making them "understand"—your spouse, your friend, your boss.

• A dream of a road that disappears into a fog or mist, a stairway that climbs but reaches no visible landing, may mean that you're not quite sure where you want to go or that you have a conflict between two different goals or destinations in life.

• A dream of flying in a plane may have to do with feelings of joy or depression. If the plane flies high, you are elated over an event in your life or over the course your life is taking. If the plane flies low, you are depressed and nervous because you are convinced you are failing.

• A dream of walking naked in a crowd means you're probably subconsciously worried you might be too honest, too open, too vulnerable.

You may or may not see yourself in any of those dreams. But looking more closely at your own dreams is worth the effort—since psychologists generally agree that dreams tell us of basic needs, desires, or fears of which we may be unconscious.

From your dreams you may find that you are refusing to deal with problems in your work or other relationships, for example. If you let your dreams bring those stresses to your attention and then do something about them, you will relieve some of those anxieties in your waking life.

You may find that your work or your home life will benefit from your dreams. The pieces of the puzzle you are trying to solve may fall into place while you're asleep.

If you've got a problem right now that you haven't been able to solve, don't just think about it with your rational, waking mind. Instead, as you go to bed tonight, tell yourself that you will find an answer as you sleep—and that you will remember the answer when you wake up. It may not work the first night, or the second. But if you let yourself "sleep on it," some morning you may just wake up with a solution to your problem.

Get more *into* your dreams, and you'll get more *out* of them. Give yourself a Feeling Fine point for paying attention to your dream messages.

Unstressing Pleasures

IT'S ALL IN THE MUSCLES

Nature gave everybody a perfect target organ for stress—muscles. They convert tension in your life to tension in your body by contracting.

The car breaks down—you clench your jaw. The roof leaks—you make a fist. The kids are noisy—you arch your back. All over your body, muscles react to stress by getting tense. And one thing is clear: when your muscles are tense all over, you're not feeling fine.

The most common headache in the world, "tension" headache, is caused by keeping the scalp muscles in a constant state of contraction. The most common cause of back pain is muscle spasm. The most common cause of eye discomfort is—you guessed it—muscle tension. Get rid of the tension in your muscles and some of the tension in your life will disappear too.

It's not hard to make muscles relax, and you don't need a biofeedback machine to do it. All you have to do is use a simple technique developed more than forty years ago by a noted physiologist, Edmund Jacobson. Dr. Jacobson is the man who taught us that the best way to get a muscle to relax is to contract it first, because nature's automatic response to contraction is total relaxation. Sound too simple? Try it.

Make a fist and clench it as hard as you can. Hold it clenched for at least five seconds, then let it go. Rest your arm and hand on your lap or a table. Let the muscles relax by themselves. See how relaxed they feel.

Try it with your face. Close your eyes, then squeeze the lids shut as tightly as you can. Hold them that way for five full seconds, then let them relax. The lids will feel so relaxed you won't want to open them.

That's the way it can be all over your body, anywhere you've got a muscle, anywhere you feel tense. You don't have to wait for a backache or a headache to start. Relax away the tension and, in time, the pain won't come.

Dr. Jacobson developed a systematic way to do these muscle relaxations. He called it progressive relaxation. There's an entire book full of the exercises he developed. Today I'll give you a few samples (we'll see more of this tomorrow). If you like the exercises you can buy the book and use this technique more often to cancel the effects of stress. Here goes.

1. Prepare by taking the phone off the hook and making sure that no one disturbs you.

2. Lie down on a bed or couch with your arms at your sides, but not touching your body. Your legs should be stretched out, but not crossed. Lie still for three or four minutes and allow your eyes to close slowly.

3. With your palms down, bend your left hand at the wrist, slowly but steadily drawing the hand backward until you feel tension building up in the back of your forearm muscles. Release the hand and allow it to drop under its own weight.

4. Rotate your left wrist so that your palm faces up. Bend your wrist and bring the hand toward you until you sense the tension accumulating in the forward portion of your forearm muscles. Then relax and allow the hand to drop down of its own weight.

5. Slowly bend your left arm at the elbow until you feel tension building in the muscles of your upper arm. Then relax, allowing the arm to fall back on the couch or bed. Repeat these procedures with your right arm.

6. Shift your attention to the left leg. Flex your ankle, drawing your toes toward you until you feel tension building up in the muscles of the calf. Let go.

7. Extend your foot so that your toes point away from you. When tension has built up in the calf, bring your toes back to the normal position. Do these same procedures with the right leg.

These exercises should leave your legs and arms feeling very relaxed. Try them to melt away tension. Give yourself a Feeling Fine point every time you do.

Eating Pleasures

THE FEELING FINE SHOPPING LIST

Supermarkets are very tempting places. Not by accident. They are made that way because the sale of food is big business. Everything is scientifically designed: the strategic lineup of foods, the height at which they are placed, the arrangement of the displays. It's all geared to create the greatest appeal and entice you into buying things—whether you need them or not.

Notice where the chewing gum and candy are located? Always near the cash register. So are the potato chips, candies, and six-packs of soft drinks. Standing in the checkout line gives you extra time to look, and before you know it you've put the candy or chips into your shopping cart.

Even without this market intrigue many foods would still be difficult to resist because they are packaged so attractively. Studies show that any time you touch a package on a shelf chances are 20 to 1 you'll buy it—even though you didn't plan to. That's why manufacturers spend so much time, money, and effort to make packages so attractive. You notice them, touch them, buy them. It works almost all the time. That's why you sometimes take home the jumbo economy size even though you live alone. That's why you may go home with bags full of fancy foods—but forget some of the essential items you went shopping for in the first place.

How do you avoid these problems? By beginning your shopping at home. That is, by making out a shopping list.

This may well be something you already do. But the Feeling Fine list is different. It has *two* columns and you use them both when you're shopping.

The first column is familiar. You use it to write down the items you need to buy.

The second column is equally important, but I'll bet your present shopping list doesn't have it. It's a space to write down the items you do *not* want to buy. There you list the things you've fallen for before that you don't want to be suckered by again—foods that contribute little to your health and provide you with little nutrition for the dollars you spend, things like soft drinks, cookies, cake, candy, and alcohol.

Your point-earning activity today, then, is to begin a shopping list, even if you're not going to shop today. Add items day by day as you think of them. The list on the next page will give you some ideas.

If you are not the shopper in your household you can still start a list and give it to the person who does

Buy More	*Buy Less*
Fresh vegetables and fruits	Heavily marbled or
Whole-grain bread and	processed meat
rolls	Candy, Cake, Cookies
Whole-grain cereal	Ice cream
Polyunsaturated fats	Pre-sweetened cereals
Chicken	Fruit in heavy syrup
Fish	Soft drinks
Tomato and citrus juices	Snack foods
Low-fat dairy products	Butter

the shopping. Use it to tell him or her which items you would like to see in next week's shopping bag and which you'd rather not see.

The Feeling Fine shopping list will help make your shopping a disciplined activity. It will also make shopping less expensive, more fun, easier, and faster. Using the list does not mean that you can never depart from what is on it; it just means that *you* control your shopping rather than being controlled by supermarket trickery. It also means that you will generally buy foods that furnish the most nourishment. Actually, with the Feeling Fine shopping list you will be freer than before to experiment with new and more interesting foods because you'll be more aware of the choices you are making.

There's one more benefit to the list. Supermarket surveys show that you are able to complete your buying in thirty minutes, on the average, if you follow a list. If you don't have a list, you're inclined to linger—and that proves to be expensive. You end up buying nonessentials which are not good for your health. And that overtime is costly in another way, since the average amount spent in a supermarket runs to about a dollar a minute.

Add more items to both sides of the shopping list and earn your Feeling Fine point for today.

Body
Pleasures

STRETCHING:
LONGER AND LOOSER

Nature gave us one spontaneous stretch we'd be better off without—the morning yawn. Have you ever had the experience of waking up and automatically going into an uncontrollable yawn? Your neck goes back as far as it will go. Your jaw goes down as far as *it* will go. Your arms go out as far as *they* will go. And—if you're as unlucky as I have been on occasion—your muscles go into spasm as far as *they* can go.

If stretching is so good for you, why does this happen? Because the connective tissues and muscles weren't *ready* to be stretched. They were in an overcontracted state. That's what happens to them when you haven't used them for a while, which you haven't when you've been sleeping. That's what happens when you're very cold.

That's why it's important to work up gradually to your stretching exercises. Don't jump out of your bed and into a stretch. Limber up first. Warm up first. Even a hot shower will help.

Doing them every day helps, too. That's why I hope you won't start today's new stretching exercises without repeating the ones you learned yesterday. As soon as you've done the old, familiar ones, get started on these new stretches.

LEG STRETCHER

1. Sit on the floor with your legs straight in front of you and slightly separated. Point your toes upward.

2. Slowly bend forward from the waist until you feel a slight stretch at the back of your legs.

3. Grasp your legs with your hands as far down as you can reach and pull yourself into the fully stretched position. Hold for 15 seconds. Try not to bend your knees. Use the strength of your arms pulling on your legs to extend this stretch, but don't overdo it.

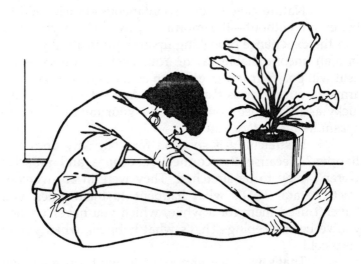

SHOULDER AND ARM STRETCHER

1. Standing straight, extend your arms over your head, with your palms facing outward.

2. Stretch your arms up and slightly to the back, breathing in as you stretch upward.

3. At the top of the stretch start to exhale.

4. Bring your arms down slowly to your sides, continuing to exhale as you do.

5. Repeat 3 times.

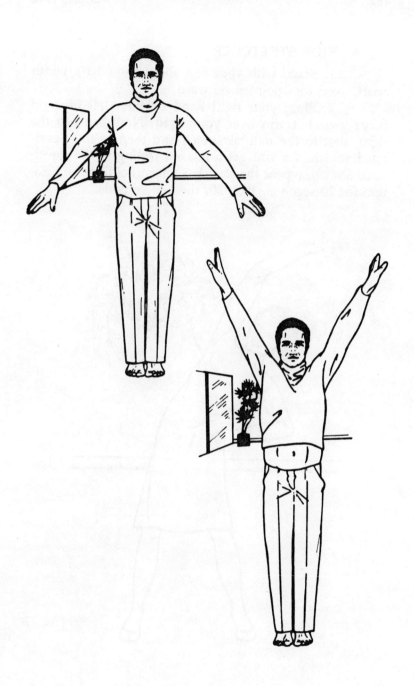

SIDE STRETCHER

1. Stand with your feet about shoulder's width apart, your toes pointed outward.

2. Place your right hand on your left hip and curve your left arm over your head. Now bend to the right, first to the natural stretch and then to the developed stretch. As you get a relaxed feeling in the developed stretch, repeat the stretch 3 times, holding the position for 10 seconds, then 20, then 30 seconds.

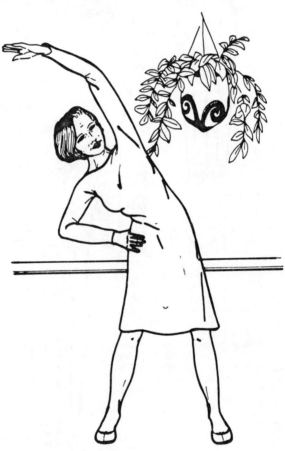

3. As a variation on this stretch, from the same standing position clasp your hands over your head. Stretch first to the right, using the strength in your right arm to pull your left arm over your head and down, and then to the left. Don't overdo it. Stay within the good feeling.

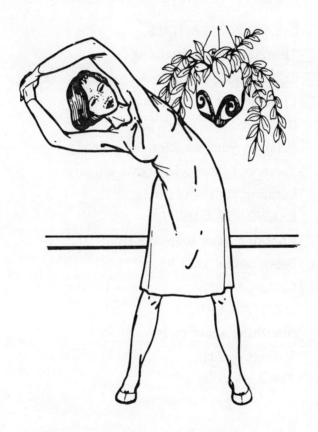

Give yourself a Feeling Fine point for trying these new stretches, and another for repeating the ones you learned earlier.

FEELING FINE POINTS
(Choose one or more from each category.)

GROWING PLEASURES
☐ **Thinking about dreaming**
☐ Taking a step toward your goals
☐ Choose your own pleasure

UNSTRESSING PLEASURES
☐ **Relaxing your muscles—completely**
☐ Vacationing through guided imagery
☐ Locating your stress triggers

EATING PLEASURES
☐ **Checking your shopping list**
☐ Being careful with liquor
☐ Cutting calories

BODY PLEASURES
☐ **Stretching some more**
☐ Limbering a bit
☐ Sharing a massage

DAY 13

Growing Pleasures

BUST OUT THE CHAMPAGNE

One of the greatest thrills in my father's life was getting a new car. What did he do the day it was delivered? He covered up the beautiful upholstery with plastic seat covers so the fabric wouldn't get dirty. For the three or four years he kept the car we'd look at and sit on those cheap, uncomfortable plastic covers. Then, when he got ready to sell the car, he'd take them off so prospective buyers could see how beautiful the upholstery really was.

We tried to convince Dad he should enjoy the beautiful cloth upholstery himself and put the plastic covers on when he was ready to sell the car, but he never bought the idea. (He finally compromised by putting clear plastic over the luxurious felt, so we could at least see the beauty of the original upholstery, even if we couldn't feel it.)

Are you making that kind of mistake—hoarding and hiding pleasures which you could be enjoying now? Which you *should* be enjoying now? Are you waiting for them to get better with age?

Fifteen years ago I bought three bottles of the best champagne in the world. I couldn't really afford them at the time, but the owner of the liquor store assured me I'd never get another chance to buy champagne like that. For fifteen years I kept those bottles, just waiting for an occasion big enough to pop the cork.

Then one day a friend told me something I hadn't known about champagne—it can spoil if kept too long. That night, with no occasion at all to celebrate, my wife and I opened the bottles one by one. Of the three, two were undrinkable and the third was just so-so.

It was a hard way to learn that the so-called treasures in life have no value if they lie unused. I'll never hoard my treasures again.

Few of the good things in life get better aging in a cellar. In fact, their value can diminish and sometimes even disappear as fashions and styles change—or as we ourselves change.

So stop hiding your treasures from yourself. It's time to bust out the champagne, even if you don't have a bottle. Your Growing Pleasure for today is to find a treasure that's been in hiding and enjoy it to its fullest.

Break out the sterling. Serve dinner to the kids on your best china. Put the milk in crystal glasses. Serve the sandwiches on your silver platter. Put candles on the table. Use the "company" linen. Why are you saving it?

Need some more ideas? Display those family heirlooms instead of keeping them wrapped up in tissue paper and locked safely away in a closet. Figure out how many times you actually wear your "best" clothes before they're out of style. Then open up your closet and wear your best outfit to work today. Or put it on when you go out tonight, even if it's not to the social event of the season.

Now is the time to put this book down and head for your own treasure chests. Don't neglect any closet, and don't forget the garage or the attic. Some of the world's greatest pleasure-treasures are waiting in those places for you to uncover and enjoy. It's time to get them out of hiding and into the open.

Find a treasure, use it today, and give yourself a Feeling Fine point for treating yourself well.

Unstressing Pleasures

ROCK-A-BYE BABY

If the unstressing techniques I've suggested in the last few days haven't solved your sleeping problems, don't give up hope. I've got more to show you.

There are two techniques which seem to help a lot of people get to sleep, no matter what their problem: repetitive action and progressive relaxation. They work especially well for people who practice them every night. You might consider trying them, even if you don't have a sleeping problem.

REPETITIVE ACTION

If you concentrate your thoughts *totally* on the repetition of a single sound, sight, or act, your body will usually relax enough to allow sleep to take over. (This is, by the way, the same kind of concentration that lies behind the effectiveness of hypnosis and meditation.) Here are some examples of how repetitive action works:

1. *Rock-a-Bye.* Lay your head on the pillow and very gently nod it back and forth. Concentrate totally on the motion of your head. The first few nights you may have to nod your head for two or three minutes before the movement lulls you to sleep. With practice you can condition yourself so well that one or two nods will be all you need to nod off.

2. *Use a Mantra.* Repeat a single sound or word aloud to yourself over and over and over again. Don't stop until you fall asleep.

3. *Use Repetitive Imagery.* Gather a flock of animals on one side of a fence and start them jumping over one at a time, counting them as they go. Yes, it's the old counting-sheep trick, but it works. If you think sheep are

a bit old hat, use cats, dogs, deer, or any other animal that makes you sleepy. Don't stop counting until you're asleep. Over the course of time you'll be counting less and sleeping more.

PROGRESSIVE RELAXATION

If repetitive action does not appeal to you, try progressive relaxation. Yesterday you learned how to do it for parts of your body, today I'll show you how to put your body to sleep one part at a time. Here's how it's done.

Start by getting into bed. Make yourself comfortable. Take a few deep—very deep—breaths. Focus your attention on your feet and your toes. Tighten up the muscles there, squeezing hard. Then let them relax. Let them go completely. Let them fall asleep.

Next, contract your calf muscles. Tightly. Bend your ankles to work the muscles in the calves. Then let go. Suggest to yourself that your ankles and calves are going to sleep.

Repeat the process with your thighs. Your buttocks. Your abdomen. One part at a time, let yourself fall asleep.

Now, move up to your fingers, your hands. Tighten. Flex. Relax. Let them fall asleep.

Repeat the process with your forearms and upper arms.

When you get to your chest, take a few more deep breaths. Slowly. Breathe in through your nose. Purse your lips and blow out slowly—slowly—very, very slowly through your mouth.

Concentrate on the muscles in your chest. Put them to sleep.

Work on your neck and head. Bend your head to the side, tensing your neck muscles. Let them fall asleep.

Finish with your face.

The entire progressive relaxation procedure should take no more than four or five minutes. The first few times you try this relaxation technique you may not fall asleep before you have gone from your toes to your head. After a few nights of practice, you won't get past your stomach before your brain—and you—are in slumberland.

What do you do if you can't sleep and nothing works for you? Not solving yesterday's problems, not planning the next day, not repetitive action nor progressive relaxation? Get out of bed! A leading sleep researcher has reported that people who lie in bed and worry because they are not asleep feel worse than people who get out of bed and putter around until fatigue finally overcomes them.

So if you can't sleep, don't waste time worrying in bed. Get up and read the paper or a magazine. Write a letter to a friend. Listen to some music. Watch television. Try to relax and enjoy yourself.

And give yourself a Feeling Fine point for working toward good sleep, the healthy way.

Eating Pleasures

SHOPPING, FEELING FINE STYLE

When you made out your double-column shopping list yesterday you took a significant step toward eating right. But neither good intentions nor a shopping list can save you from some of the other shopping traps that await you.

Here are a few things that get people into trouble when they shop:

- They go to the market hungry and buy things they don't really need. Surveys show that hungry shoppers not only buy 20 percent more food than they ordinarily would, but they also buy the "wrong" kind—foods high in calories that need no preparation and can be consumed immediately.
- They take the kids along and get pressured into putting things into their shopping carts they wouldn't dream of buying if they were by themselves.
- They buy the "giant economy size," which seems to be a bargain. It isn't if you can't eat it all.
- They use food coupons to buy things they never wanted in the first place.

Here are some tips to help you protect yourself from these traps.

1. Never shop when hungry. If necessary, eat a snack before you leave the house.

2. Shop alone. Leave the kids at home or with a neighbor.

3. When there are different-sized packages of the same product do some unit-pricing. Check the cost per ounce or pound to avoid paying more for large-sized boxes. Buying in quantity saves money only if you don't have to throw out spoiled food or eat extra helpings just because it's there.

4. Ignore food coupons for items you really don't need.

5. Check the specials in newspaper ads before you go shopping.

6. Always read nutrition labels on packaged or canned products to get the most for your money.

7. Check open dating if it is used where you live. This date is stamped on the carton or container to tell you the date by which the product should be used.

8. Stay clear of aisles packed with cookies, chips, sodas. Don't walk down them and you won't be tempted to buy what's in them.

Before you get to the cash register, do a Feeling Fine cart check—check your cart and ask yourself:

1. Did I buy nutritionally inappropriate foods? (Did I buy that big bag of pretzels because the kids were along?)

2. Did I buy more than I needed? (Does the jumbo box look like too much?)

3. Did I buy something I didn't really need? (Do I really have to have that hamburger supplement just because I have a food coupon for it?)

If the answer is yes, return the item. Replace the large "economy" size for a smaller, more economical one. Return the empty-calorie food and choose something better. Put unnecessary items back on the market shelves where they belong—rather than on your kitchen shelves where they don't.

It is never too late to return something, even if the cashier is already ringing up the sale. Tell the checker you changed your mind. Adjustments can always be made.

For every shopping suggestion you follow today (or whenever you go to the market) give yourself a Feeling Fine point.

Body
Pleasures

STRETCHING:
NOW THAT YOU'RE LIMBER

It's not hard for the tension in your life to become the tension in your muscles, because muscles are a natural target organ for stress. The more stress you get, the more your muscles contract. If you've got stress all the time, they'll stay contracted all the time. When they stay contracted all the time, they begin to hurt.

As we saw in Day 12 of Unstressing Pleasures, contraction of muscles in the face and scalp is the most common cause of headaches. But we've also seen that the head isn't the only place in the body that suffers pain because of muscle tension. Many people translate the stress of their life into tension in their back or neck muscles. Some pick on the muscles of their arms or legs. But wherever the tension lies, the solution is the same—the muscles must be relaxed.

A great way to get a muscle to relax well is the tensing techniques you're already familiar with—progressive relaxation. Another way to achieve the same effect is to stretch it as far as it will go (without pain). Presto —total relaxation will follow.

Today we'll continue with more stretching exercises. This time I'd like you to concentrate not just on how the muscles feel when they're being stretched but also on how they feel when the stretch is over. You'll see how relaxed they become—and how good they feel—as they return to their natural state. You'll also see how you can use stretching to get rid of tension no matter where it is.

Before you do the new exercises, give the familiar ones another try. I'll bet you find you can already stretch farther after just a couple of days of practice. Before you do anything—don't forget to warm up.

THE TOE TOUCHER

As you get started with this toe toucher it may help if you set a pile of books in front of your feet. If you can't reach your toes at first, there'll be something in front of you that you *can* reach. Make the pile thinner and thinner as you become more and more flexible.

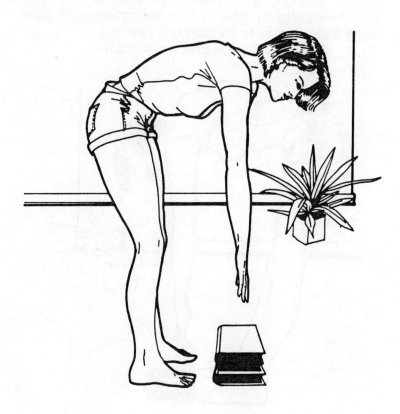

1. Stand with your feet about 4 to 6 inches apart and your toes pointing straight ahead.

2. *Slowly* bend forward at the waist, letting your arms and neck hang loosely. When your body comes to a natural rest position, you may feel the pull anywhere from your neck to your heels, but particularly at the calves and the backs of your thighs.

3. Slowly, gradually, stretch your fingertips a little closer to your toes and hold the position for 10 to 15 seconds. Never, never bounce your body to get your fingers down farther.

4. As you get up from this stretch, always bend your knees slightly first to take the pressure off your lower back. Return to the standing position.

5. Repeat this exercise *slowly* 3 times.

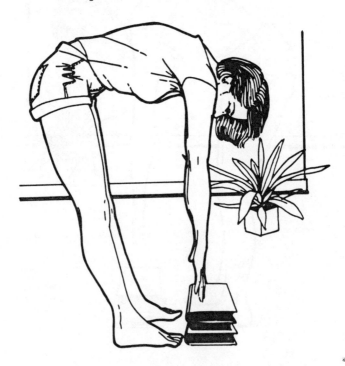

THE CHEST STRETCHER

1. While standing hold firmly onto both sides of a doorway. Your hands should be behind you at approximately shoulder level.

2. Lean forward with your chest and head up. Hold for 5 to 10 seconds.

3. Repeat 3 times.

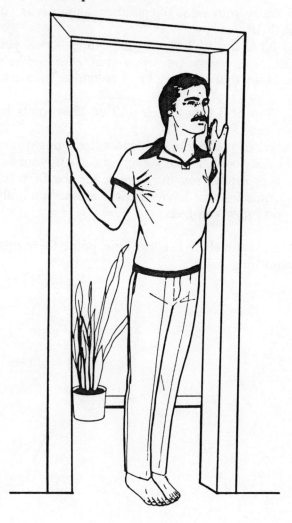

THE FACE STRETCHER

1. Sit down in a comfortable position.

2. Open your mouth wide. Wider. Relax it.

3. Raise your eyebrows as high as you can. Higher. Relax them.

4. Open your eyes as wide as you can. Let them close.

5. Raise your ears. Wiggle them as much as you can. Relax them.

6. Now do it all at the same time—open your mouth, raise your eyebrows, open your eyes and raise your ears. Hold that position for 5 seconds. Then relax *completely*.

7. Repeat 3 times. Relax 10 or 15 seconds between each time.

8. When you're done, spend at least one minute with your eyes closed, relaxing every muscle in your face and scalp completely. You may notice for the first time how many muscles you have in those areas. You'll also see how good they can feel.

Give yourself a Feeling Fine point for getting into the stretching habit.

FEELING FINE POINTS
(Choose one or more from each category.)

GROWING PLEASURES
☐ **Enjoying a treasure**
☐ Achieving a goal
☐ Reaching out with appreciation
UNSTRESSING PLEASURES
☐ **Moving into sleep**
☐ Returning stress to its rightful owner
☐ Watching your target organs
EATING PLEASURES
☐ **Shopping smart**
☐ Cutting sugar
☐ Choose your own pleasure
BODY PLEASURES
☐ **Stretching some more**
☐ Enjoying a walk
☐ Massaging yourself

DAY 14

Growing Pleasures

GUIDED IMAGERY FOR PROBLEM SOLVING

Until now we've used guided imagery for fun and relaxation. Today I'm going to show you another way to use it—for problem solving. It really works, and there's a good reason why.

The human brain is divided into two hemispheres. One hemisphere functions completely at a verbal level. It constantly processes words. The other hemisphere operates at a visual level. Pictures and images are its forte (dreams probably play themselves out in this part of the brain). However, the visual hemisphere, despite its penchant for pictures, can also deal with complex thoughts just as well as the verbal hemisphere can.

Under normal circumstances, when you grapple with a problem you deal with it on the verbal side of the brain. On the verbal side you approach the problem very logically—and very slowly. In the long run you generally come up with an answer, but it takes a lot of time to solve a problem using the word side of the brain.

Brain researchers don't really know why a strictly verbal solution is slow to develop. But they think that a word-oriented problem-solving process may be too methodical. First you have to find the right words to formulate the problem. Then as you consider various solutions—discarding some, retaining others—in each case you must think of the words that will state each solution correctly. If you can't find the right words, sometimes you never find the right answer.

The visual side of the brain, for reasons not clearly understood, seems to deal with problems in a more straightforward and faster way. It comes up with solutions you never would have dreamed of just by using the verbal side.

How can you get in touch with this problem-solving machine? You can do it by discussing your problem with your creature-adviser, the one you met in one of our earlier discussions of guided imagery.

Are you getting the feeling that this creature business has gone a little too far? Trust me. I really haven't gone off the deep end. There are sound, scientific reasons for using your creature in this way.

By working on a problem with your creature-adviser, you are in essence bringing the visual side of your brain into the problem-solving process. The animal, of course, is nothing more than a symbol for your inner self, and talking to the animal amounts to talking to yourself, but on a brain wavelength you don't often use.

Recently I used my own personal creature—a rabbit named Corky—to solve a work-related problem I had. For days I had been trying to seek a way out of the situation. No solutions. Lots of frustration. Lots of stress. Then one day I thought, "Let's see what Corky has to say about this."

I closed the door to my office, drew the blinds, and sank into my chair. Quickly I imagined myself at my relaxation spot—a ski slope at Mammoth. Within seconds Corky popped up. I stated my problem and asked him, "What should I do?"

"*You* shouldn't do anything," the rabbit answered unhesitatingly. "Let Frank handle it. That's not your problem."

Why hadn't I thought of that? It was the right

answer, although it had escaped me for days while I pondered the problem.

I got on the phone to Frank (who handles administrative matters for my television show) and told him about my conversation with the rabbit. Frank agreed to take care of the problem. Within seconds I felt better.

I'll admit the solution should have been obvious all along. But that's just the point. It wasn't obvious to the verbal side of my brain. Only when I called in my creature-friend was I able to move into a fresh area for the solution.

Are you ready to give it a try? Here's how to use the technique:

Take precautions against being disturbed. Make yourself comfortable. Now think of a problem you've been trying to solve. In your mind's eye go to your place of relaxation and find your creature-adviser. Say hello. Then, no matter how silly it seems, ask the creature to help you with the problem. Pose the question and listen for an answer. It will come.

More often than not your adviser will give you a matter-of-fact solution. No rationalizations. No excuses. You may not always like the response you get. You may even want to argue with your adviser. Go right ahead.

Talk to your creature and you'll be tapping a voice of inner wisdom. Frequently you will be able to follow that voice's advice simply, immediately, and with a rarely felt sense of rightness.

Of course you don't have to do something because an imaginary animal tells you to, but at the very least you'll find it worthwhile to listen to what the animal has to say.

Give yourself a Feeling Fine point every time you try to solve a problem with guided imagery.

Unstressing Pleasures

PATIENT, HEAL THYSELF

Today you're going to learn to quiet your stomach, slow your heart, lower your blood pressure, and dull your pain. In other words, you're going to learn how to start healing yourself.

That's a strong statement coming from a man who was taught in medical school that those things couldn't be done. Stomach contractions, heart rate, and blood pressure were supposed to be regulated by the autonomic (meaning "automatic") nervous system. They were supposed to be beyond our conscious control. That's what we medical students were told.

Here's what they didn't teach us. That Indian Yogis could suspend their breathing and slow their pulse rate. That men could walk on coals without burning their feet and lie on beds of nails without bleeding. That concentration could make headaches go away. And they never taught us about a German neurologist named Schultz, who refused to believe that autonomic functions were beyond voluntary control and developed a program called "autogenics" to prove it. During the next three days you'll see how autogenic exercises work and you'll get a chance to try them yourself.

When there's no way to escape stressful situations, autogenic exercises may give you the ability to deal directly with your stress target organs. Autogenic exercises may be the thing that keeps your pulse from racing, your head from throbbing, or your stomach from hurting. When there's no way to avoid the stress, autogenic training may be the thing that saves you from pain and cancels your stress.

There's nothing new about autogenics. The Yogis didn't know it, but they were practicing a form of autogenics. The men who walked on burning coals weren't aware of it, but they were doing autogenics, too. So were the hypnotherapists who made pain disappear. Underlying all of their techniques is the same basic activity—concentration. Total concentration. In hypnosis it's total concentration that makes your body receptive to the suggestions presented. In meditation it's total concentration on a mantra that makes your body achieve a state of perfect relaxation. In autogenics it's total concentration on the exercises that makes your body react the way it does.

It's not that total concentration will put you in full control of every physiological function in your body, but it will help you achieve deep relaxation and reduce the effects of stress on your target organs.

During the next three days you'll see how autogenics works. Today we'll start with a simple demonstration of how a single body function—control of blood flow to the skin—can be affected by an autogenic exercise.

Normally if you held the bulb of a thermometer tightly against your hand the reading would be around 90 or 91 degrees, because the temperature there is cooler than it is inside your body. Sending more blood to the skin will make it warmer. So if our autogenic exercise for today is working, you'll know it because the temperature of the skin on your hand will rise.

Are you ready? Find a thermometer and we'll start the exercise. Follow these instructions.

1. Sit down in the most comfortable chair you can find. Put both hands in your lap. Grip the thermometer firmly between your thumb and first two fingers, but not so tightly your hand gets tired. If you wish, tape it to your thumb or use some tape to hold the bulb between your index and third fingers.

2. Relax and wait until the thermometer has a chance to reach the temperature of your skin—about five minutes. Read the temperature. (*Note:* not all thermometers go as low as 90 degrees. If your medical thermometer doesn't, any ordinary household thermometer will do.)

3. Next, close your eyes and relax as much as you can.

4. Concentrate on the hand holding the thermometer. Imagine that the hand is beginning to get warm. In your mind's eye, make a picture of the hand filling with blood. Pretend your fingers are filling up with warm, red blood, and that as they do, the space between the fingers is getting smaller and smaller, until the fingers are touching.

5. Repeat the images in your mind for ten minutes. Imagine your hand getting heavier and heavier with blood. Feel it get hotter and hotter. Concentrate intensely on these ideas. If anything interrupts or distracts you, just bring your mind back to your hand.

6. After about ten minutes open your eyes and read the thermometer again. Chances are good that more warm blood will have shifted to your hand and the reading will be several degrees higher than when you started.

Don't be discouraged, though, if the temperature doesn't go up. Sometimes it may even go down. It may simply take more concentration. And sometimes it just may not work.

So what does changing the temperature in your hand prove? For one thing, it shows that through mental processes you can alter the way your body functions. Once you are convinced of that, a host of illnesses and physical complaints come under your conscious control.

For example, warming the hands is growing in popularity as a way of stopping migraine headaches. By turning on the blood flow to their hands and turning off the blood flow to their heads, migraine sufferers are learning to get their headaches under control.

Let me tell you about another unique way it can be used—one I learned from personal experience while skiing. My wife, Priscilla, and I were waiting our turn to get on a ski lift when I realized I had lost my gloves.

"Are you going back to try to find them?" Priscilla asked, casting a nervous glance at the long line stretching ahead of and behind us.

I was torn. If I walked all the way back to the village to look for my gloves, I'd lose an afternoon of skiing. Yet how could I ski barehanded in below-freezing temperatures?

"Well," said Priscilla, somewhat mischievously, "you're supposed to be so good at controlling your body temperature, why don't you 'will' your hands into staying warm?"

I had no choice but to accept the challenge. As we rode to the top of the mountain I worked on my hands, literally thinking "warmth" into them. I skied comfortably without gloves for the rest of the afternoon.

Don't leave your gloves behind when you go skiing. Do give yourself a Feeling Fine point for giving autogenics a try.

Eating Pleasures

WHERE DO YOU EAT?

Discarded cups. Torn candy wrappers. Rusting cans. Flip-top rings. Everyone's complaining about the effect of our eating habits on the environment. Why doesn't anyone pay attention to what the environment does to our eating habits?

I never eat popcorn—unless I'm at the movies. I never eat dessert at home—until I fill the dining room with company. I never take a second drink—unless I'm at a party. Bread and butter? Not for me—except on an airplane. Pastries? Never touch 'em—except when I've got time to kill in the doctors' lounge at the hospital.

The fact is, there's something about some environments or situations that makes us eat even when we're not hungry. Sometimes it's just because the food is there. Sometimes it's because others are eating. And sometimes it's because the food is really tempting, and that's the only place or time we can get it.

If you respond to these environmental and situational stimuli every time they are present you end up eating a lot more than you really want—or need—to. Here are some examples of how to control yourself in those situations:

Movies. Plan ahead. Don't wait for the junk food at the counter. Treat yourself to a sensible dessert at home before you go, or take one with you to the theater, such as dry-roasted nuts, raisins, or a small can of fruit juice.

Dinner Parties. Eat slowly. While others are on second helpings you will still be on your first.

Bakeries. Do you pass a bakery going to or from work that tempts you inside? Take another street. If you must go in, buy bread or rolls instead of cake and cookies.

Office Coffee Breaks. Do you find it hard to skip snacks during the coffee break? Then skip the coffee break instead. If you must have coffee, bring a thermos; then you won't have to pass the food in the cafeteria line. Change its name to a Pleasure Break, and make it a different pleasure every day. Try walking or reading, stretching or limbering, instead of eating.

Kitchen. Don't snack if dinner isn't ready. Try some delaying tactics by keeping your hands and mind busy: write a letter, walk the dog, play a game, strum a guitar, knit a sweater, take a shower.

Dinner-Table Leftovers. Don't let the sight of uneaten food be the problem. When the meal is over clear the table right away. Put leftovers in opaque containers or foil wrap, not the see-through kind. Then when you open the refrigerator or cupboard you'll see containers, not things to eat. Also make foods hard to reach by putting tempting foods on a top shelf so that you need a kitchen stool to reach them. Or wrap them up well and put them in the refrigerator behind other items.

Aftertastes. Get rid of tempting tastes in your mouth. They make you want to eat more. Substitute the taste of toothpaste.

The best way to become aware of and then neutralize situational stimuli at home is to eat in only one room and in one place in that room. Let's call it your "eating place."

This means you don't sit in front of the TV in the bedroom or living room and munch. You don't walk around the house with food. You don't nibble while you cook. You don't hold the refrigerator door open and snack.

If you really want to eat and you are not at your eating place, go there. Take with you only as much food as you really want to eat. Then sit down and eat it. There. Nowhere else.

Okay, pick your eating place. To help mark it, make yourself a placemat, but not an ordinary placemat. You should write the following on it: I ONLY EAT HERE. WHEN I AM HERE, I ONLY EAT.

Write this with a felt-tip pen on an old placemat or a paper one. Set it up in the one place in your home where you usually eat. Then, when situational stimuli come up, ask yourself, "Do I want to eat badly enough to interrupt what I'm doing, get the food, and take it over to the eating place?" Most often the answer will be no.

After you have made the choice consciously several times you will begin to make it without giving it much thought. You will free yourself from the stimuli that lead you to food you do not need and don't really want.

You won't have this placemat around forever, but you will retain the lesson you've learned from it.

Become aware of the situational stimuli in your life that cause you to do extra eating. Devise a technique for gaining control over them and earn a Feeling Fine point every time you take charge of your eating habits.

Body Pleasures

FELDENKRAIS: MOTION WITH MOSHE

If you're sitting down right now (which most people do when reading), hold onto this book with both hands. Keep reading, but stand up for a moment. Do it now, and then sit down.

A simple motion. Or was it?

According to Moshe Feldenkrais, an Israeli physicist, who has devoted the greater part of seventy-five years to studying the human body and mind, it was anything but simple. To stand up, you unnecessarily tightened the muscles at the back of your neck, pulled your head back, tightened your chest muscles and, finally, moved the muscles in back of your knees to straighten up your legs. If you don't believe that try it again.

Such complicated motions are fairly typical, Feldenkrais believes, of the way we go through life: in a series of tense and often superfluous movements that, in the aggregate, interfere with our ability to feel well—physically, psychologically, and emotionally.

Accordingly, Feldenkrais has worked out almost a thousand different exercises (some with forty variations) to re-educate the body. The exercises are not meant to build strength or endurance but to increase awareness of the body, to loosen it up, enabling you to make movements gently and easily, with a minimum of effort and a maximum of pleasure and efficiency. In the process, Feldenkrais maintains, people will become more sensitive, not just to themselves but also to the world around them and the way they relate to their environment. He also maintains that these movements will help people become more supple and limber, which means that they are less likely to strain or hurt themselves in sports or daily activities and less likely to get backaches and other muscle pains. It's an interesting idea—one worth trying.

Because of space limitations, I am offering only one exercise, which is especially beneficial for the back and hamstrings. Feldenkrais's book, *Awareness through Movement*, describes many more in detail. If this exercise makes you feel good—as it did me—you might want to try others from his book.

By the way, the first time I read through this exercise I didn't want to do it. It looked like it would take a long time. And, frankly, I thought I'd feel a little foolish. But I did it and I liked it. Put aside your inhibitions and give it a try. No one's watching. (You'll enjoy it more if you wear comfortable clothes in which you can easily stretch and move.)

Here we go (reading aloud helps):

First of all, stand with your feet together and bend forward to touch your toes. See how far you can reach. Do this only once, but remember how close you came to your toes and what it felt like in your back and legs. Then return to a standing position.

FIRST MOVEMENT

Stand with your legs comfortably spread apart (approximately the same distance as the width of your shoulders). Place your right hand on the outside of your upper right thigh and gently caress downward, using a circular motion. As you stroke downward bend your right knee and raise your right heel off the floor, shifting your weight to the ball of your foot. Then caress upward, letting the heel go back down to the floor and allowing your right leg to straighten.

While you are caressing downward, let your head and upper body move forward and to the right. Notice your breathing. Try breathing in through your nose when you are standing up and out through your mouth as you caress down the leg.

Do this caressing movement on the outside of your right thigh 5 or 6 times, always doing it slowly and gently and *not* trying to force yourself to reach as far down your leg as possible. In fact, do less than you are capable of doing. Don't stretch or strain. Stop before you get tired. Let the movements be easy and pleasurable.

Now walk around a bit and see whether your right side has some new sensation.

SECOND MOVEMENT

Stand with your legs spread comfortably apart as before. Place your left hand on the inside of your upper right thigh. Caress down the inside of your right thigh with the left hand, bending your right knee and lifting the right heel as you stroke downward. And as you caress upward let your knee straighten and your heel go back to the floor.

Again, do the movement slowly and gently, without trying to stretch. You will find that your hand gradually slides farther down your leg without any extra effort. The slower and more gently you do the movements, the faster the improvement. Breathing out through your mouth as you caress down the leg also makes the movement easier, since muscles relax more during exhalation.

After doing this movement 3 or 4 times, let the right hand caress the front of the right thigh at the same time, so that now the right hand caresses the outside of the leg and the left hand caresses the inside of the leg.

Allow your head and upper body to move forward and to the right and your pelvis to the left as you caress down the leg.

By now you may be reaching all the way to the calf or even the ankle without consciously pushing yourself to do so.

After a few movements like this, again stand up and walk around. See whether you notice any more difference in feeling between your right side and your left.

THIRD MOVEMENT

Stand with your feet spread apart as before. With your right hand on your right buttock, caress down the back of your right leg, using the same circular motion used in the other movements.

Bend your right knee and shift your weight to the ball of your foot as you caress down the leg. Move up and down the leg 5 or 6 times, letting your head and torso move forward.

After a few movements let your left hand also caress down the front of the leg so that now you are caressing the front and back at the same time.

Return to a standing position and walk around the room. Notice any differences between how the right and left sides of your body feel. You may find that your right side feels lighter and more buoyant, longer and smoother than the left side.

FOURTH MOVEMENT

Stand with your feet spread comfortably apart and close your eyes. Place your left hand on the outside of your upper left thigh. Now focus your mind on your left leg. Don't move. Instead, imagine that you are doing the same caressing, bending, and weight-shifting movements on your left leg that you actually performed on your right leg. In your mind's eye picture your right hand caressing the inside of your left leg at the same time that your left hand caresses the outside of your left leg. Spend about 3 to 5 minutes just thinking through the various movements you did.

Now open your eyes and actually caress down your left leg. After you have imagined performing the exercise, you will probably find that when you begin caressing your left thigh you will be able to go all the way down to your left ankle almost immediately, without much effort. Having done the exercise in full on the right side, merely *thinking* about the movements in relation to your left side will loosen you up sufficiently to help you move freely along the whole length of the leg. But the technique works only with movements you have already experienced in detail.

LAST STAGE

Stand with your feet together and reach down to touch your toes. You may be pleasantly surprised to find your back muscles and hamstrings more limber than they have been in years.

As you can see there is no stretching or straining with the Feldenkrais method, no strenuous movements. Once you have performed the exercise, the next time you can *think* yourself through it. Move the muscles (mentally) just as though you were actually doing the exercise. Then when you actually perform the exercise again, the body does not have to push as hard and can go still farther.

If you have just been *reading* the directions, go back and start following them. Then give yourself a Feeling Fine point for finding another healthful Body Pleasure.

FEELING FINE POINTS
(Choose one or more from each category.)

GROWING PLEASURES
☐ **Consulting your advisor**
☐ Breaking a taboo
☐ Choose your own

UNSTRESSING PLEASURES
☐ **Finding out about autogenics**
☐ Relaxing your muscles—completely
☐ Easing stress with guided imagery

EATING PLEASURES
☐ **Taking control of your eating cues**
☐ Adding to your Feeling Fine shopping list
☐ Choose your own pleasure

BODY PLEASURES
☐ **Enjoying new movements**
☐ Giving your back some support
☐ Choose your own pleasure

DAY 15

Growing Pleasures

HABITS: FINDING YOUR TRIGGERS

Not too long ago, after an eight-year abstinence from cigarettes I suddenly found myself smoking heavily again. When I took the time to think things over, I recognized a pattern to my smoking. I was smoking frequently where I had not smoked before—in my car. I couldn't understand this new compulsion to smoke behind the wheel. Driving wasn't stressful to me—I enjoyed driving. Yet, almost automatically and almost always at the same spots on the road I was lighting up cigarettes on my way to and from work. One day I decided to find out why.

I turned the car around and drove back to the point where I had reached for the cigarettes. There was my trigger—a big billboard with a woman in Levis urging me to smoke Winstons. Something about that woman made me smoke. Something in her looks, her gaze, her pose, was making me reach for a cigarette.

It wasn't accidental. The advertising agencies spend millions developing ads like that one. They put them everywhere they can to make suckers out of us— cigarette suckers.

That lady was my *cue* to smoke. She never said it out loud. She didn't need to. She knew exactly how to tickle my subconscious so I'd want to smoke.

I'll bet most of you have some cues that play an important part in your life, too—cues that make you do unhealthful things by habit.

Don't get me wrong. Habits can be helpful. It's nice to be able to get the little things in life done without having to think about them each time; things like picking up your purse before you leave the house or remembering to take the keys out of the ignition before you lock the car. But when it comes to habits like picking up a cigarette, taking a drink, or swallowing a tranquilizer, you're talking about habits that don't help you at all. Those habits are hazardous to your health—sometimes hazardous to your family and friends.

A single cigarette won't kill you, but a pack a day for forty years may. An occasional drink doesn't make a drunk, but too many drinks make an alcoholic. Even a tranquilizer now and then, at a time of great stress, probably does no harm. But too many tranquilizers make a dull, depressed person.

Most people who smoke *can't* stop at one. Many people who drink *must* keep filling the glass. And some people who use tranquilizers put pill after pill into their mouths without even thinking about it. For them, smoking, drinking, and pill taking are no longer deliberate acts. They have become thoughtless, compulsive, repetitive behaviors—habits that are inherently hazardous.

Of course, not everyone reading this chapter has these problems. Unfortunately, though, statistics show that half of the people reading this book are smokers, two out of five take two or more drinks a day, and one-fifth have already swallowed their daily tranquilizer.

If you don't smoke, drink, or take pills too much, I've got a present for you—a Feeling Fine point. Give yourself one point now, whether or not you finish reading this section. You deserve it. (However, if you do read on and find a way to apply some habit-breaking principles to another behavior you'd like to stop—excessive worrying, too much anger—give yourself another point.) The rest of you—the smokers, heavy drinkers,

and chronic pill takers—will have to read further. You'll
have to start finding out what triggers your unhealthy
habits.

Don't expect to be able to come up with all your
cues right away. You'll have to think about them. More
often than not, you're not fully aware of the cues that
make you act the way you do. But when you become
more aware of these "triggers" and the role they play in
your habit patterns, those habits become much easier to
break.

Is it Sammy Davis? When he lights up during a
show do you have to light up, too? When they pour the
beer in the commercial, do you have to head for the refrigerator? Is tossing and turning before you are able to
fall asleep your cue to reach for the Valium?

Today's task is to start identifying the cues that
"turn you on" to unhealthy habits. (Then, during the
next two days we'll talk about the way to turn these unconscious and unwanted responses off.)

Take a look at the list of common cues to smoking, drinking, and pill taking that follows. If you find
some things on the list that trigger you into action, write
them down on a piece of paper or mark the appropriate
boxes. Then add some of your own cues to the list.

☐ TV commercials
☐ Billboards
☐ Ringing telephones
☐ Being late for
   an appointment
☐ Coming in the front
   door after work
☐ Getting stuck in traffic
☐ Having to pay bills
☐ Cocktail hour
☐ Coffee break

☐ Sitting down with
   the morning paper
☐ A hot drink at the end
   of a meal
☐ Seeing someone else
   light up
☐ Being alone
☐ Watching the news
☐ The arrival of a visitor at
   your home or office
☐ Facing a pile of work

If reading the list leaves you blank, then you've got more work to do. To earn your Feeling Fine point for today, for the next twenty-four hours you're going to have to keep a diary. Every time you reach for a cigarette, a drink, or a pill—*before* you put it in your mouth you've got to identify the trigger, or cue, that made you act. You'll not only be finding the cues to your habits, you'll also be discovering the first key to breaking them.

Give yourself one point for every cue you discover.

Unstressing Pleasures

AUTOGENICS: BREATHING

You don't need cold hands to appreciate autogenic exercises. All it would take to make you an avid autogenic advocate, as I am, is one session with my friend Dr. Norman Shealy. Norm is a neurosurgeon turned holistic healer and one of the nation's experts on pain control. He teaches autogenic exercises to his patients so they can learn to control their pain. But he doesn't stop there. He says these exercises are the best way to "rebalance" your nervous system, to cancel the effects of stress on your body. I've used his exercises, and I find them to be the most relaxing ones I've ever tried.

My wife and I use Norm's recorded exercises in our home. His voice is so relaxing, so hypnotic, that we're unable to listen to them in bed without falling asleep. The only way we can hear the end of the tape is to get out of bed and listen with the lights on. They work better than any sleeping pill I ever heard of, and there's no hangover afterward.

Norm's complete program is contained in his book, *90 Days to Self-Health*. He has recorded some of the exercises from the book on audio cassettes, so the sound of his voice is as near as your mailbox. There's no better way, in my opinion, to get the feel of an autogenic exercise than to hear Dr. Shealy's tapes. But I didn't want you to have to wait for a tape to try the exercise, so he gave me permission to print part of his program in this book. Space limitations make it impossible to include even one entire exercise, so I've done a little editing and excerpting.

The one for today focuses on breathing, because breathing correctly is a key step in achieving complete relaxation. That's your goal with the exercise today—relaxation.

You'll need some help. It isn't possible to read the instructions and follow them at the same time. Either get someone to read the exercise to you as you do it, or read it yourself into a tape recorder and then perform the technique as you play back your cassette.

Before you start, find a quiet place and make sure you won't be interrupted. Make yourself comfortable in a chair, close your eyes, and concentrate intensely on everything you hear. Now here's the exercise:

> I am not listening to anything from my mind or anything said. I listen to all the noises occurring in the world around me. I listen.
> *(Leave a two-minute pause on the tape so that you can listen.)*
> I notice that listening intensely for every sound but not reacting to it, withdrawing my thought processes from it, is actually a way of distracting my body and mind from their spontaneous activities.

By concentrating intently upon each little sound,
by focusing my attention on such a narrow
aspect of the total possible sensation outside
myself, I slow myself down.

As I really listen carefully, listening for everything occurring outside myself, I am at rest.

I listen again. I hear. I am aware only of sounds
outside myself. Any time I have a thought,
any time I think about going off on a vacation or anything pleasant or anything bad,
I focus my attention again on sound, just
sound.

*(Pause two minutes—leave a two-minute pause on the
tape.)*

Now I will concentrate only on my breathing. I
breathe as deeply as I can comfortably, all
the way in and all the way out, for one minute.

*(Breathe deeply for one minute—leave a one-minute
pause on the tape.)*

I take maximum deep breaths in and maximum
deep breaths out and count the number of
times that I breathe.

*(When you record the tape, count twelve breaths,
twelve very deep breaths—and leave a pause that
length on the tape.)*

I have completed twelve breaths. That is twelve
breaths per minute. I was perfectly comfortable, perfectly relaxed.

I concentrate not upon my own thoughts about
breathing, my own apparent needs. But I
just breathe purposefully at the rhythm suggested.

Slowly I breathe in and hold it for ten seconds. I
don't force it. *(Pause ten seconds.)* I breathe
out, slowly.

I breathe in, slowly in. I keep stretching a little
  deeper. Now I breathe slowly out. I breathe
  in. Slowly and deeply I breathe in.
I start another breath out. I breathe in. Breathe
  out.
(Count one breath every fifteen seconds.)
I breathe in. I breathe out.
My body breathes itself.
I focus all my mental energies only upon breath-
  ing. I am aware only of breathing.
(Count one breath every fifteen seconds.)
I breathe in. I breathe out.
I take deep, deep breaths.
I breathe in, I breathe out. I breathe in. I breathe
  out. I breathe in. I breathe out.
I allow my body to breathe itself but as it does I
  concentrate on each breath.
I feel the air coming in and the air going out,
  freely and comfortably.
I focus upon breathing and feeling my breathing.
  I am only breathing.
(Now repeat.)
I am relaxed and comfortable.
I am relaxed and comfortable.
I am relaxed and comfortable.
Each time I practice these exercises I benefit
  more and more.
Every day in every way I am becoming more and
  more healthy.
(End of exercise.)

Find a reader or make your tape. Give yourself
another Feeling Fine point for making these arrange-
ments. Learn to control your breathing with autogenic
exercises and you'll be amazed at how relaxed you can
feel.

Eating
Pleasures

WHY DO YOU EAT?

7:30	Breakfast. One pancake left over. Didn't want to waste it. Ate it.
9:00	Arrived at office. Had coffee with cream and sugar.
10:30	Coffee break. My day to bring the pastry—two for everybody. I'm no cheapskate.
12:00	Lunch. Bought a hot fudge sundae. After all, I left six French fries on my plate.
1:30	Took deposit to bank. Stopped for a candy bar.
2:30	Argument with fellow worker over air-conditioning temperature. Ate the candy bar.
3:00	Cheese cake.
4:00	Chewed a piece of gum.
4:30	Meeting—coffee again.
5:30	Stopped off for a drink.
6:30	Prepared dinner. Sampled the spaghetti and garlic bread. Had another drink.
7:00	Dinner.
8:00	Picked up date for bowling. Ate handful of nuts while waiting.
8:30	Bowling. Had some beer and pretzels.
11:00	Worried about meeting tomorrow. Couldn't sleep. Watched late-late show. Had small dish of ice cream.

Why do people eat? For survival? To get energy? To keep going? Take another look at the diary above. It's an eating diary I had one of my staff members keep one day. He eats often, doesn't he? He's not the only one.

Surveys reveal that every day the average person eats three regular meals—and six or seven snacks. And that's just the average! The heaviest snackers were children up to age 12 and women between 25 and 44. They had up to twenty food contacts a day! We seem to be a nation of nibblers.

Take another look at my staff member's diary. Two other things besides hunger inspired his extra consumption of food: (1) situational stimuli and (2) emotional upsets.

I wrote about situational stimuli yesterday—things like the candy counter at the movies and the peanuts on the bar, which remind us to eat even though we may not actually be hungry. That's one problem you see in the diary.

The second problem is the use of food to cover up emotional upsets. Anger, nervousness, guilt, worry, frustration, depression, loneliness, and boredom become cues to try to satisfy ourselves with food. Instead of tackling the problem, we tackle the cheese cake.

This use of food to alleviate situational urges and emotional distress is often unconscious. How, then, can we distinguish between them and true hunger?

One way is to localize your hunger. If you feel hungry in your *stomach* you are probably really hungry. But if you are eating because your *mouth* seems to be asking for something, the temptation to eat probably has nothing to do with real hunger.

If you're not sure where the "hunger" is, you've got to ask *why* it's there. The crucial moment to ask that question is before your fingers actually touch the target food. At this point it's not too late to back off, to short-circuit the whole action. And you can do this by asking one question each time before you eat: "Why do I want to eat?"

If the answer is "I am eating because I am hungry," fine. Sit down and eat.

If the answer is "I am eating because the food is there" or "because that sure smells good" or "because I didn't get that party invitation" or "I'm just a little nervous and I'll feel better if I eat," then stop. There are better ways of handling the situation.

Today I want you to try two things. First I want you to keep a diary—just like my staff member did. To make it easy for you, we have included a sample diary page. Every time you eat anything (candy, nuts, cheese, fruit, milk, a regular meal, even gum) stop and ask yourself *why* you ate. Check off the appropriate column. At the end of the day you should have a rather good idea of the drives that keep you eating and eating and eating. You will see—perhaps for the first time—just how many times you eat when the cue is not hunger itself.

Be sure to save the diary. You will refer to it tomorrow.

The key to stopping these unconscious urges to eat is simple—bring them to your conscious attention. To help you do that we've prepared a poster for you bearing that critical question: WHY DO YOU WANT TO EAT?

Why a poster?

So you'll be reminded to ask yourself that question again and again. One suggestion never does anybody any good. That's why God carved the Ten Commandments in stone instead of just whispering them into Moses' ear.

Want to earn a quick Feeling Fine point? Cut the poster out. Make several more like it. Tape one onto every door that stands between you and food: refrigerator, freezer, pantry, cupboard—even on food containers that are in plain view, like cookie jars and see-through canisters. It may not be subtle, but if it works, who cares? Give yourself a Feeling Fine point for every one you put up.

REASON FOR EATING

FOOD

	Hungry	Bored	Angry	Habit	Nervous	Depressed	Courtesy	Lonely	Other

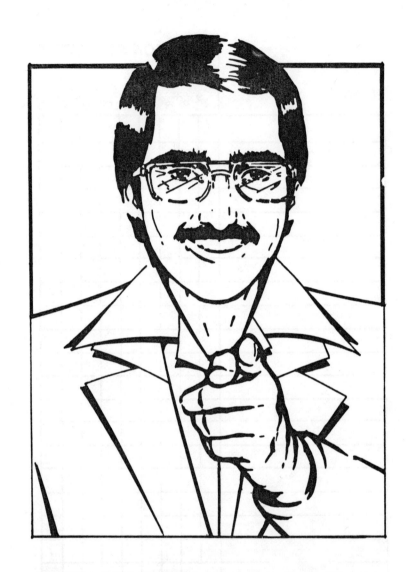

WHY DO <u>YOU</u> WANT TO EAT?

Body
Pleasures

ISOMETRICS:
MUSCLES WITHOUT MOTION

In the 1950s a group of West German physiologists caused quite a stir when they announced that strenuous exercises such as running, weight lifting, and push-ups were not necessarily the best way to develop the human body. Instead they recommended "isometric conditioning exercises" which produced static tension—a high state of tension in a selected muscle for a brief period of time. The tension could be produced anywhere, anytime, by such maneuvers as gripping a table and squeezing or by clasping hands and pressing. It was a tensing of one set of muscles against either another set of muscles or some immovable object. Repeated several times, it was claimed, the tension would increase muscle strength. Are they any good?

Isometrics can't do everything. They will not whip a sagging and long-neglected body back into robust condition. They will not do anything for joints, heart muscles, lungs, or the blood system. But, when done along with other exercises, they can help increase the strength of individual skeletal muscles.

If you'd like to see how isometrics work, try the following exercises. You may want to incorporate some of them into your total body-pleasuring program. But as you do these exercises maintain the tension no longer than *eight seconds*. And, as I've said for all the other exercises, start easily. Work up very gradually to maximum effort.

LEGS AND ANKLES

1. Sit at a desk or table and grip a wastebasket between your ankles.

2. Lift up your legs, squeezing the basket between your ankles. Hold it tightly at least 6 to 8 seconds. Return it to the floor.

CHEST

1. With your back straight, sit in the middle of a doorway with your body parallel with the jambs and your legs crossed.

2. Place one hand against the jamb where it meets the floor. Push hard against the jamb. Hold for 8 seconds. Repeat with the other hand.

3. Grasp both jambs a little higher and bend your elbows. Push hard. Hold for 8 seconds.

4. Raise your arms as high as they will go. Press your hands against the jambs. Hold for 8 seconds.

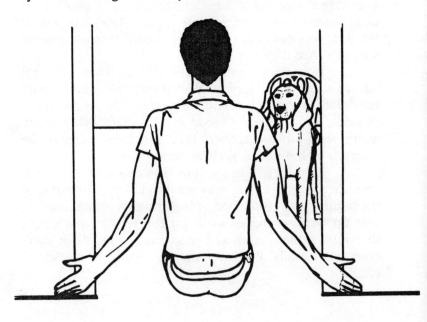

THIGHS AND CALVES

1. Stand with your back about 10 inches from a wall or door jamb.

2. Lean the upper portion of your body against the support.

3. Slowly lower yourself into a sitting position with your thighs parallel with the floor.

4. Maintaining that position, try to lift your heels as far off the floor as possible. Hold for 8 seconds.

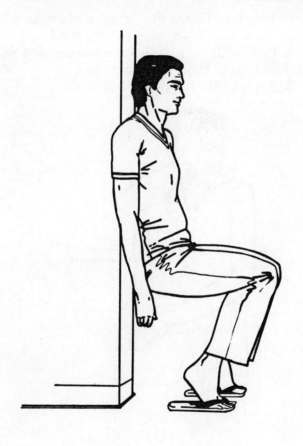

BACK, SHOULDERS, UPPER ARMS

1. Lie on your back with your legs stretched out and your arms at your sides.

2. Keeping your hands, head, and heels flat against the floor, try to lift your pelvis and legs off the floor. The body's weight is on your shoulders. Hold for a count of 8. If you're not successful the first time, try again tomorrow.

NECK

1. Turn your face to the right and place the palm of your left hand on the left side of your head.

2. Push with your left hand while resisting with your head and neck. Hold for 8 seconds.

3. Repeat with the right hand.

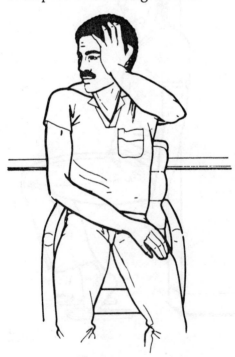

One nice thing about isometrics is that they can be done very quickly and are no-sweat exercises. You can do some of them in your office at your desk or while waiting on line or for the light to change.

Try them. You'll like them. Give yourself a Feeling Fine point when you do.

FEELING FINE POINTS
(Choose one or more from each category.)

GROWING PLEASURES
☐ **Finding your habit cues**
☐ Spending $1 for fun
☐ Choose your own pleasure

UNSTRESSING PLEASURES
☐ **Breathing autogenically**
☐ Removing yourself from stress
☐ Choose your own pleasure

EATING PLEASURES
☐ **Counting the times you eat**
☐ Handling liquor with care
☐ Skipping calories

BODY PLEASURES
☐ **Building muscles**
☐ Stretching muscles
☐ Massaging muscles

DAY 16

Growing Pleasures

HABITS: BREAKING THE CHAIN

Finding your cues isn't enough to break a habit. Cues are just the first link in a chain of behaviors that, when taken together, make up what we call a habit. If you really want to break the habit, you're going to have to break the chain first. How? Several ways.

1. *You can remove the cue from your environment.* For example, if watching people smoke in your office makes you want to smoke, you could ask them not to light up when they're in your office. Don't be bashful. Put a sign on the door. If they ignore your sign, don't ignore their smoke—ask them to put it out.

Of course, this technique won't work when you're in someone else's office. Usually the person who "owns" the territory gets to make the rules. So try removing the cue when you can, but don't count on this technique by itself unless you plan to spend the rest of your life as a hermit.

2. *You can remove yourself from the environment that contains the cue.* If people won't stop smoking in the employee lounge, you should stop visiting the lounge. Then you won't be tempted to join them for a smoke. The trouble with this technique is that you can't always take yourself out of the picture. If you have to go through the lounge to get to the bathroom, you haven't got much

choice. Don't give up on this technique. Just don't count on it to do the entire job.

3. *You can "break the behavior chain" that the cue begins.* There's an old saying that a chain is no stronger than its weakest link. The saying applies to the chain of events that make up a habit, too. If you want to break a habit, start with the weakest link in the chain. Where is it? It's that part of the chain that is farthest from the final activity. Let's use smoking to show you how the technique would work.

Smokers not only have a smoking habit (very strong), they have a lighting-up habit (strong), and a cigarette-carrying habit (not quite so strong), etc. Attack the weakest part of the habit chain and you will find it the easiest part to break. For example, if you have a cigarette in your mouth and a match in your hand, the chance of your not smoking is very small. If you have a cigarette in your mouth but you don't have a match, your chance of not smoking is better, because now you have to find a light before you can smoke. If you don't have a cigarette in your hand, your chances of not smoking are better still, because now you need not only a match but a cigarette, too.

It's easy to see how this works with eating. You have a much better chance of not snacking before you go to bed if you don't leave your bedroom than if you stand in your robe in front of an open refrigerator. It's easier to break the habit of going into the kitchen than to break the snack habit once you get there.

Of course, it isn't always easy to find the weakest link in your own behavior chains or to put the theory into practice. But even under these circumstances there are still other ways to make breaking habits easier.

4. *You can interrupt the chain.* Break up your usual sequence of events. Take the habit out of your habit. Give yourself time to think. Give yourself a chance to change.

The following tips and tricks are specifically designed to help you interrupt habits like smoking, drinking, and taking tranquilizers. But you'll find they also work for almost any behavioral pattern you want to change. Use them and help yourself break the habit chain.

CIGARETTES

To fortify your battle with cigarettes try the following:

• Keep only one pack of cigarettes around you at any given time, and don't keep that pack in its usual place. Put it in different pockets than you usually do. Put it in different parts of the house when you are at home. If you make it difficult for yourself to get at a pack, you'll become aware of every cigarette you smoke.

• Don't carry cigarettes with you *at all*. If you want to smoke you'll have to bum your cigarettes from friends, acquaintances, fellow workers. You'll suddenly realize how frequently you smoke. Chances are you won't ask too often—and you'll be smoking less and less.

• Don't carry matches or a lighter.

• After each smoke get up and wash the ashtray. Then put it away somewhere so that you'll have to make the extra effort to go look for it the next time you light up.

ALCOHOL

Behavioral tricks also work well with alcohol:

• Keep only one bottle of your favorite drink at home, and keep it in an inconvenient place. Pour only one drink at a time, and put the bottle back after you have poured.

• If you find yourself drinking a great deal at parties, it may be that you simply need to do something with your hands. Okay, have a drink, or even two. But then spend the rest of the evening holding a glass without liquor. Even if the glass only has water in it, it may serve as the anxiety-diminisher you need.

• If you are invited to dinner and you know there will be a protracted cocktail hour before dinner is served, arrive late so that you have time for only one drink.

• If you are giving a dinner party, cut your cocktail hour in half. (And be sure to wait to have a drink yourself until the guests arrive.)

TRANQUILIZERS

Even tranquilizers can be cut down with behavioral tricks:

• Make them hard to reach. Don't put them in the medicine chest. Keep them on the highest shelf in the kitchen, where you'll need a stepladder to get to them.

• Wrap a dish cloth around the bottle with rubber bands. Every time you want a tranquilizer you'll have to prolong the time needed to get to it—maybe just enough to convince yourself that you don't really need it.

• Put tape on the cap. Every time you think you want a pill you'll have to struggle with the tape to get to it.

• If you carry a pillbox with you when you go out during the day, put only one tranquilizer in it to last you for the time you are away from home.

What's the point of all this trickery? To make you look before you leap. To give you time to break the chain. To force you to ask yourself, "Is what I'm about to do really necessary?" Try the tricks and see if they don't work for you. You'll have another well-deserved Feeling Fine point for breaking the chain.

Unstressing Pleasures

AUTOGENICS: WHOLE-BODY RELAXATION

From hand-warming to breathing control to total body relaxation—that's what autogenic exercises are all about. Not only can they be used to control specific body functions, but they are also superb for producing deep and total relaxation.

The nice thing about autogenics is that the more you practice, the easier it gets to do. After awhile neither a friend nor a tape recorder is necessary. The routine becomes so familiar that you can play it back in your mind just by closing your eyes and concentrating. Do it often enough and you'll be able to use autogenic exercises almost anytime, anywhere: in the den during the day, in the bedroom at night, in the yard, at the office, even in the doctor's waiting room.

And the more you use them, the better they'll work. The more you use them, the faster they'll work. If you use them enough, you'll soon become "conditioned." You'll be able to achieve many of the effects just by cueing yourself with key words.

A few words of caution, however. You're not going to master autogenic techniques in a few minutes or even a few days. Reading a condensation of the exercises is not the same as being taught by Norman Shealy. His patients are successful at controlling their pain with autogenics, but some of them spend *hours* each day doing the exercises.

We're not suggesting that you spend hours a day doing autogenics. We're not recommending that you use it to treat serious medical problems. We are saying that it's a great way to cancel stress and "rebalance" your system.

Today we'll try another cut-down version of one of his exercises. Once again you'll have to record the exercise or get someone to read it to you while you do it. Remember, to make it work you'll have to concentrate completely on every word in the program. Today's exercise is designed to produce general relaxation.

Begin by lying quietly in a comfortable position, arms and legs uncrossed. Now, here's the exercise for today.

> I take a deep, slow breath.
> I hold my breath and slowly exhale.
> I take another deep, slow breath.
> I hold my breath and pull my toes toward my head, tightening my leg and calf muscles.
> I feel the tension.
> I breathe out and let go completely.
> I take another deep, slow breath.
> I hold my breath and make a fist with both hands, tightening my arm and shoulder muscles.
> I feel the tension.
> I take a deep, slow breath.
> I hold my breath and tighten every muscle in my body until I feel my whole body start to tremble with tension.
> I breathe out and let go completely.
> I take another deep, slow breath.
> I hold my breath and tighten every muscle in my body.
> I hold on to the tension.
> I breathe out and let go completely.
> I take another deep, slow breath.
> I hold my breath and tighten every muscle in my body.

I hold the tension.
I breathe out and let go, relaxing completely.
I concentrate on slow, deep breathing through-
    out this entire exercise.
I feel very calm and quiet.
I feel very comfortable and quiet.
I am beginning to feel quite relaxed.
I am beginning to feel quite relaxed.
My feet feel heavy and relaxed.
My ankles feel heavy and relaxed.
My calves feel heavy and relaxed.
My knees feel heavy and relaxed.
My thighs feel heavy and relaxed.
My hips feel heavy and relaxed.
My legs feel heavy and relaxed.
My hands feel heavy and relaxed.
My arms feel heavy and relaxed.
My shoulders feel heavy and relaxed.
My neck feels heavy and relaxed.
My jaws feel heavy and relaxed.
My forehead feels heavy and relaxed.
My whole body feels heavy and relaxed.
My breathing is getting deeper and deeper.
I can feel the sun shining down on me, warming
    the top of my head.
The top of my head feels heavy and warm.
The relaxing warmth flows into my right shoul-
    der.
My right shoulder feels heavy and warm.
My breathing is getting deeper and deeper.
The relaxing warmth flows down to my right
    hand.
My right hand feels heavy and warm.
The relaxing warmth flows back up to my right
    arm.
My shoulders feel heavy and relaxed.
My neck feels heavy and relaxed.

My jaws feel heavy and relaxed.
My forehead feels heavy and relaxed.
My whole body feels heavy and relaxed.
My breathing is getting deeper and deeper.
I can feel the sun shining down on me, warming
    the top of my head.
The top of my head feels heavy and warm.
The relaxing warmth flows into my right shoul-
    der.
My right shoulder feels heavy and warm.
My breathing is getting deeper and deeper.
The relaxing warmth flows down to my right
    hand.
My right hand feels heavy and warm.
The relaxing warmth flows back up to my right
    arm.
The relaxing warmth spreads up through my
    right elbow into my right shoulder.
My right elbow, my right shoulder feel heavy
    and warm.
The relaxing warmth flows slowly throughout
    my whole back.
I feel the warmth relaxing my back.
My back feels heavy and warm.
The relaxing warmth flows up my back and into
    my neck.
My neck feels heavy and warm.
The relaxing warmth flows into my left shoulder.
My left shoulder feels heavy and warm.
My breathing is getting deeper and deeper.
The relaxing warmth flows down to my left hand.
My left hand feels heavy and warm.
The relaxing warmth flows into my heart.
My heart feels warm and easy.
My heartbeat is calm and regular.
The relaxing warmth flows down into my
    stomach.

My stomach feels warm and quiet.
My breathing is deeper and deeper.
The relaxing warmth flows down into my thighs.
My thighs feel heavy and warm.
The relaxing warmth flows down into my legs.
The relaxing warmth flows up through my right
    calf, to my right knee, to my right thigh.
My legs feel heavy and warm.
My breathing is deeper and deeper.
The relaxing warmth flows slowly up through
    my left calf, to my left knee, to my left
    thigh.
My breathing is deeper and deeper.
My breathing is deeper and deeper.
The relaxing warmth flows up through my ab-
    domen, through my stomach and into my
    heart.
My heart feels warm and easy.
My heart pumps relaxing warmth throughout
    my entire body.
My whole body is heavy, warm, relaxed.
My whole body feels very quiet and very serene.
My whole body feels very comfortable and very
    relaxed.
My mind is still.
My mind is quiet.
My mind is easy.
Nothing exists around me.
I am comfortable and still.
I feel an inward peace.
I feel a new sense of well-being.
My entire body and mind are in perfect
    harmony.
Every day in every way I am becoming more and
    more healthy.
(End of exercise.)

Do autogenic exercises every day and—in every way—you will feel better and better. You'll have another point every time you do.

Eating Pleasures

KEEPING THE SOLUTION FROM BECOMING THE PROBLEM

I've never been able to keep my troubles a secret from my wife. In the old days, when I was a smoker, she knew without asking whenever something was bothering me. How? It was the only time I'd light up at home.

I don't smoke anymore, but she's still sharp at spotting the times when things aren't going right for me. She doesn't even have to be in the room with me. She only has to listen for the refrigerator door. Whenever I'm at the refrigerator to get food between meals or after dinner she knows I'm trying to satisfy some stress or problem with food.

Look at the eating diary you prepared yesterday. How many times did you use food as a substitute solution for another problem? Did you find yourself reaching for a snack because you were irritated and needed something to make you feel better? If so, take a closer look at the role emotions play in your eating patterns.

Any stress can trigger a food craving. People under stress can finish a full dinner and still eat all night long. But eating all night long won't make them feel better.

When a craving has nothing to do with hunger, food will never satisfy it. When a problem has nothing to do with hunger, food will never solve it. In fact, if you keep putting things in your mouth whenever something goes wrong, food itself becomes the problem.

What can you do about these emotional urges?

The next time you find yourself at the refrigerator or cupboard door, read the little poster you've put up. Ask yourself, "Why am I eating?" If it is not because you're really hungry, close the door on the food and give some thought to attacking the real problem. Here are some approaches.

Take the edge off your fury, not off a chicken wing or cheese sandwich. The best solution is often the most direct one: deal with your anger or frustration or depression, because that is where the cause of the problem lies. Talk or write to the person with whom you are having the difficulty and try to clear the air.

Sometimes you can't deal with the problem directly. If this is the case, try doing something physical to dissipate the feeling. Use some of the activities in the Body Pleasures section of this book: take a walk, do some stretching, try five minutes of breathing exercises.

Substitute another pleasant activity for eating. Pleasure your hands, your eyes, or your ears. Turn on the stereo, go out to a movie or a concert, talk to your best friend about your feelings.

Or use some ideas from the Unstressing section: try the progressive relaxation technique, do five minutes of guided imagery, use the autogenic exercise.

If you're bored, neutralize the problem by going to a sporting event or a play. Organize a family game, do a jigsaw or crossword puzzle, play backgammon with a friend. Or absorb yourself in a magazine or book. Do something you like, even if it takes time. In the long run it will be easier to make up the time than to lose the extra weight you'll put on if you give in to your urge to eat.

By the way—if you can never seem to answer the question of why you are eating and feel that your snacking is due to some "mysterious compulsion," you might contact an organization called Overeaters Anonymous. Patterned after Alcoholics Anonymous, it has more than 700 chapters around the country offering members a supportive environment in which to solve their mutual compulsive eating problem.

For every time you spot and neutralize an emotional eating cue, give yourself a Feeling Fine point.

Body Pleasures

THE BATH AND SHOWER: WASH YOUR TROUBLES AWAY

When it comes to bathing, we have thrown out a lot of good things along with the bath water. For many people the pleasure is gone. It's time to bring back the joy and make bathing the experience it can be, not just a way to wash off the dirt.

Remember when your parents told you not to spend so much time playing in the tub? Now that you're grown up you can—and should. It's time to play again. The bath is another place to come in contact with the feelings in your body.

The pleasures can begin the moment the tap water is turned on. Tune your ears into the sounds of the rushing water. Add some music from your stereo or radio.

Settle down with a good book. (A bath pillow is nice, but not necessary.) No reason why you can't have a glass of wine, a cup of tea, or some hot broth while you're just lying there. Read, sing, or just do nothing but let yourself relax in the warm waters. Enjoy the environment.

Don't rush. There probably aren't too many places more pleasant than where you are. Take a five- or ten-minute soak. Don't rush out because the water gets cold. If the water gets too cool, turn on the hot-water tap again. When you're ready lather down, but don't use your hands. That comes later. Use a wash cloth, a rough-textured loofah sponge, or a bath brush. These will slough off dead skin and stimulate your circulation. Use a pumice stone to smooth out rough surfaces on the feet and elbows. Lather well all over.

You've already learned about self-massage. Try it in the tub. The sudsy water makes the movements easier and creates quite a different feeling than when you massage with dry hands.

Pleasure your skin. Stroke every inch you can reach. Gently. Firmly. Feel your body come alive.

When you are ready to step out of this kind of bath, many of the kinks and tensions of the day will disappear down the drain along with the bath water.

After the bath make your skin really come to life. Rub down with a thick towel.

If you don't have a tub, your shower can also give you many of the body sensations and satisfactions that a tub gives, especially if you use one of the massage or needle-spray shower heads now available commercially.

The shower is also a great place to do some of your stretches or limbering exercises, but only if you have a nonslip surface.

If you have both a tub and a shower, don't feel that using one eliminates the other. Many a devoted bather will take a shower to get clean and a bath right after just for the pleasure and relaxation that is available in the tub.

Take enough time to treat your body right under water, and earn yourself another Feeling Fine point.

FEELING FINE POINTS
(Choose one or more from each category.)

GROWING PLEASURES

☐ **Breaking the habit chain**

☐ Enjoying a hidden treasure

☐ Paying attention to your goals

UNSTRESSING PLEASURES

☐ **Relaxing with autogenics**

☐ Talking to your companion

☐ Choose your own pleasure

EATING PLEASURES

☐ **Keeping your emotions off your hips**

☐ Shopping smart

☐ Choose your own pleasure

BODY PLEASURES

☐ **Bathing for pleasure**

☐ Walking for pleasure

☐ Choose your own pleasure

DAY 17

Growing
Pleasures

THE SCS PLAN AND HABITS

I don't have anything against cigarettes, alcohol, or tranquilizers. It's what they do to your body that bothers me.

I'm not going to tell you to throw away *all* of your cigarettes, pour *all* your liquor down the drain, or dump *all* your pills in the toilet. As I said before, one cigarette won't hurt anyone, nor one drink. (I can't say that about tranquilizers because one single tranquilizing pill can do you in if you suffer a side reaction to it.)

Usually the damage these things do to your body is the result of taking too much. A pack a day for forty years and you've got emphysema—if you're lucky. (The unlucky ones get emphysema in *twenty* years and lung cancer in forty.) One pint a day and you've got alcoholism—if you're lucky. (The unlucky ones also get bankruptcy, divorce, and cirrhosis of the liver.) One prescription a month and you've got dependency—if you're lucky. (The unlucky ones get depression.)

What's the answer? Part of it you learned yesterday—lowering the dose through breaking the chain. Another way to lower your dose is with the SCS Plan. The same thing that works for overeating works here: *Skip, Cut,* and *Substitute.*

One nice thing about substituting is you don't waste a lot of time on the old pattern. If you decided you wanted to learn how to speak French, you wouldn't try to unlearn English first. You would simply try to make the French word come out instead. Initially that's difficult, but if you work at it long enough it will come as naturally as speaking English. Meet a friend on the street and presto, without stopping to think you say "bonjour" instead of "hello." In the same way you can learn to substitute a new behavior for the one you want to get rid of.

We'll show you how SCS works with habits, and you can start using it now.

CIGARETTES: SKIP

Smoke only the ones "that count." If you don't feel you *must* have it, don't smoke it. Using the chain-breaking techniques such as keeping your pack far away from your fingertips will help you greatly with this one.

CIGARETTES: CUT

Smoke only the first half of each cigarette. Put it out while it's still long. You get far more of the cancer-causing tars in the second half, anyway. Whenever you buy a new pack take all the cigarettes out before you smoke one. Mark the halfway point on all of them with a felt-tip pen and put them back in the pack or box. Then, when you're smoking each one, stop as soon as you reach the mark and throw the rest of the cigarette away.

CIGARETTES: SUBSTITUTE

Try to figure out what urge the cigarette you're reaching for is going to satisfy. Then substitute a less harmful solution. Are your fingers longing to hold something? Give them a pencil to hold and let them doodle. Does your mouth desire something? Try sugarless gum or a carrot stick. Is it simply stress? Get up and walk it off. Run it off. Whatever you do, don't try to smoke it away. That doesn't work.

ALCOHOL: SKIP

Try to eliminate every other drink you would usually take. If you feel better holding a glass, pour nothing but mixer in the glass every other time. Add some ice cubes, a slice of lemon or lime, and carry the glass wherever you go. Sip it slowly and you'll never know the difference.

ALCOHOL: CUT

Reduce the dose by putting only half as much liquor in each drink. Use a tall glass. Fill it to the top with mixer and ice cubes and you'll think you're getting twice as much as before.

ALCOHOL: SUBSTITUTE

Drink for flavor instead of effect. Try a Virgin Mary (tomato juice alone) instead of a Bloody Mary. If you really like the flavor of the liquor you've been drinking, you don't have to drink alcohol to get it. You can actually buy extracts of most liquors. The extracts contain all of the flavor and few of the side effects. Try them with your favorite mixer.

TRANQUILIZERS: SKIP

Try facing the world without anything. You will survive! You may be a little shaky, but take my word for it, you will survive. Get yourself ready for it. Put on your best clothes, your best face, and give it a go. After a few tries you'll probably find it's nice to see the world with clear vision.

TRANQUILIZERS: CUT

Halve the dose. Cut each pill in half. Take half, flush half. Halving the dose does not double your trouble, it cuts your habit in half. And it's not half as hard as you think.

TRANQUILIZERS: SUBSTITUTE

This is the time to call on one of the relaxation techniques that you've learned. Use visual imagery to visit your relaxation spot. Look up your advising creature and have a chat. Meditate. Do something good for your nervous system and it will treat you more kindly in return.

Use the SCS plan to lower your doses of cigarettes, alcohol, and tranquilizers, and give yourself a Feeling Fine point for each try.

Unstressing Pleasures

THE RELAXATION RESPONSE

Back in the 1960s a new cult materialized on the American scene. The common denominator for its members was the practice of transcendental meditation—TM. Its devotees said transcendental meditation could wash away the tensions of modern society and bring the practitioner to a special state of physical and psychological tranquility.

Word of the promise of TM spread and centers popped up near every college campus. What had been a small cult mushroomed into a major movement as more and more people sought to learn the secrets of TM—at $75 and later $125 for the course.

Here's what they got for their money. They got the chance to bring some fruit or flowers as an offering of devotion to the Maharishi, who formulated the movement in this country. They got to hear a lecture about his philosophy and teachings. All that out of the way, they were then given a secret "mantra"—a sound, they were told, which would help carry them off to that state called "transcendental meditation."

It was only a matter of time until the technique fell under the skeptical scrutiny of research workers. Many thought that they could disprove the "nonsense" that this white-robed guru from the East was passing off on the gullible. Into the labs they went, measuring alpha waves, pulse rates, blood pressure, and anything else that could be counted. Much to their surprise they found that TM practitioners were indeed capable of bringing themselves to a state of tranquility.

Dr. Herbert Benson of Harvard University, for example, found several changes that could be measured in volunteers who meditated in his laboratory. Oxygen consumption, he learned, decreased 10 to 20 percent during meditation. Lactate, a chemical produced by the skeletal muscles, dropped in meditators. Other physiological activities, including heart rate and brain-wave activity, also slowed during meditation. All in all, the Harvard researcher concluded, when people meditate a new and distinctly measurable state of tranquility sweeps over them. Dr. Benson called these physiological changes the "relaxation response."

One of Dr. Benson's most important conclusions: achieving the relaxation response is not dependent upon a protracted ritual. You don't have to pay a tuition fee, you don't have to place an offering on an altar. You don't even have to get a secret mantra to achieve the relaxation response—you can make up your own. And you can learn the meditation technique at home if you're willing to practice and be patient. During the next three days we'll describe the technique for you so that you, too, can use meditation to cancel some of the stress in your life.

Let's start now. Follow these simple rules.

1. Get comfortable. Pick a quiet place, preferably without bright light, and find a comfortable chair to sit in.

Close the door, take the phone off the hook, and tell everyone around you that you do not want to be interrupted—*for anything!* With experience you'll be able to concentrate in a wide variety of situations, but beginning meditators should pick an environment free of distractions.

2. Close your eyes and allow yourself to relax. You can't force yourself to relax—you must let it happen. Try a few deep breaths, some guided imagery, or whatever turns you *off* the best. Let every muscle go limp.

3. Start repeating your mantra. You can try the word Dr. Benson suggested ("one"), use the "universal mantra" ("ummmmmm"), or make up your own mantra. If you decide to use your own, try words with "s" or "sh" sounds in them. Most of the $125 mantras my friends have bought at TM centers have such sounds (some people just can't keep a secret): shush, shireen, shurah, shah, seesaw, shesaw.

Whatever the sound, keep saying it over and over and over again. Say it to yourself or, if you prefer, whisper it out loud. Again and again and again and again. As you repeat it concentrate totally on the sound of the word.

4. Hear nothing but the sound of your mantra, if you can. Most people can't do it. The world is so full of noises and the mind so full of thoughts, that sooner or later (probably sooner), your concentration will lapse and you'll find that you're thinking of something other than your mantra. You'll hear a car. Someone in the next room will make a noise. You'll think of a bill you forgot to pay.

At first you may get upset about the distractions. Don't get angry with yourself. Don't judge how well you're doing. Don't try to force your mind back to the mantra. That doesn't work. Instead, simply accept the fact that you've drifted and concentrate on the mantra again. Do that until, once again, you are concentrating totally on the mantra.

Repeat the gentle process of returning to your mantra every time you lose concentration. If nothing else, this exercise will make you more aware of all the distractions which tug at your mind and clamor for your attention every minute of the day. No wonder you're stressed!

5. Keep at this activity for ten minutes. It will seem like forever. Don't keep checking the clock. Your own internal clock will tell you when the time is up. If you don't trust your internal clock, ask someone to call you after ten or fifteen minutes. Don't be afraid to meditate a few extra minutes.

6. After your ten minutes are over, return to "the world" slowly. Stop repeating your mantra but keep your eyes closed for another minute or so. Allow your thoughts to poke their way back into your mind. Then open your eyes and return to your normal activities.

Don't expect a miracle. If you have simply been able to concentrate on your mantra most of the time, you will have done well. It's going to take many practice sessions before you reach the "special state" everyone talks about. One thing you *can* expect is to be relaxed when it's over.

That's all there is to the technique, but it's not quite as simple as it sounds. You must be willing to practice it again and again, or all you'll achieve is relaxation. That's not bad, but it's not as much as meditation has to offer.

For today let's not worry about the "special state." Just try the technique once as described and you've earned yourself a Feeling Fine point for taking ten minutes to relax.

Eating
Pleasures

HOW YOU EAT: ENJOY! ENJOY!

For several days I've been telling you what not
to eat and what to do when you *shouldn't* eat. Today it's
time to talk about what to do when you *should* eat. I can
sum it up in two words:

Enjoy, enjoy!

Eating should be an enjoyable sensory experi-
ence, and not just for the sense of taste, either. It's possible to pleasure every sense during a meal—if you try.
Pleasure your nose with good aromas. Pleasure your eyes
with attractive dishes. The more you pleasure all of your
senses while eating, the more satisfied you will feel when
you get up and walk away from the table. You'll find
yourself eating less and enjoying it more. Here's how it's
done:

1. Don't start eating until you've done something to put your worries aside. Nervousness and irrita-
tions interfere with digestion. Before you eat spend just
two or three minutes with one of our relaxation techniques. Or, if you have the opportunity, take a ten- or
fifteen-minute walk.

2. Take a complete break for every meal, even if
it is only a brief one. Devote that small amount of time
completely to eating. To concentrate fully on the joy of
eating there should be no other distractions. Don't hunch
over reports or letters with a sandwich. Don't watch TV
while you are eating. Give all your attention to one activity or the other.

3. Sit down when you eat—no eating on the run.

4. Don't allow interruptions during a meal.
Modern conveniences like the phone can also be distract-

ing. If you get a call while you're eating, take the number and call back when you're through. Relish your eating first.

5. Eat slowly. We often put our meals away so fast we barely recognize what we are eating—or even that we have eaten at all. Take your time and savor your food.

6. Chew your foods deliberately. Enjoy their consistency. Cut every bite into small pieces. Make your usual cut, and cut it in half again. Enjoy its aroma. Give your tongue time to taste every mouthful. It's not only good table manners but it's healthful as well, because digestion begins in the mouth, where carbohydrates start breaking down.

7. If the first portion was adequate, don't have a second helping.

Meals are marvelous times for bringing people together to communicate. It's a great time for a family, sometimes the only time. In my house we find meals are a great time to review everyone's day: what the kids did in school, what my wife and I did at work, and what lies ahead the next day for all of us.

What about those of you who live alone? Since many of you don't want to be alone with your food, the most common thing you do is turn on the TV at mealtimes. It's a companion, a presence. If turning on the set during dinner makes you feel pleasurable and happy, there's nothing wrong with that. All I ask is that your eyes leave the screen (or the page, if you are reading) when you are about to put a bite into your mouth. Focus instead on the food. If you don't, the distraction of television or reading may make you eat too fast and, as a result, too much.

Give yourself a Feeling Fine point for enjoying, enjoying as you eat.

Body Pleasures

ENDURANCE: GETTING TO THE HEART OF THE MATTER

When I was growing up Charles Atlas was America's ideal of physical fitness—the strong man with bulging muscles rippling across acres of chest. During recent years, however, our concept of physical fitness has changed. Now we are concerned with a much more important muscle—the muscle of the heart.

As we all know heart disease takes a fearsome toll. Even women, once seemingly immune to heart attack, are becoming almost as vulnerable as men in their later years. But you don't have to sit back and wait for a heart attack to strike you. You can strike first and prevent it from happening.

When you are under stress—especially the physical kind—you need more oxygen to meet the additional demands of your tissues. To fill that need the heart beats faster and harder to pump more oxygen-bearing blood to the critical areas. If the heart muscle is weak and flabby, the blood supply will be inadequate and the heart will fail under the increased load.

To feel really fine you need to increase the capacity and efficiency of your heart to pump blood and distribute oxygen. You need healthy and lean heart tissues and muscles. You need a heart conditioned to withstand greater stress or greater activity without pushing you to the threshold of exhaustion. To give yourself a heart with sufficient endurance to handle all the demands made on it, it's vital for you to undertake a heart-strengthening program.

What can you do?

Start by reducing the number of cigarettes you smoke. By keeping your blood pressure at a normal level. By eliminating excessive saturated fats from your diet. By diminishing tension in your life.

Equally important, you can increase your heart's ability to endure stress by making it a more efficient and enduring organ.

The only way to strengthen a muscle—any muscle—is to make it work harder for a while. How do you do that with the muscle of the heart? Exercise, of course, but not just any kind of exercise. Walking, limbering, stretching, even calisthenics will not keep the heart in fine form. These exercises may force the heart to work a little harder than normal, but they won't make it work hard enough to build endurance.

Let's demonstrate this right now. First, let's measure your normal heart rate, and then perform a few simple exercises to see how they affect that rate.

To find your normal rate take it when you are rested and relaxed. Put your forearm, with hand palm up, on a table. Take the first three fingers of your other hand and place them about a half inch from the top of your wrist. Then press gently into the sinews of your wrist at that point until you can locate the pulse beat.

Now, keeping your eye on a watch with a second hand, count the number of times the pulse throbs in a 30-second period. Each throb is equivalent to one heart beat.

Multiply the number of throbs by two to arrive at the number of heart beats per minute. Write that number down so you can remember it. (In the average person, the heart at rest beats from 60 to 80 times a minute, although the normal range is wider than that.)

Now perform one of the following activities (do all of them if you can):

1. Do your limbering and stretching exercises for the day.
2. Take a five-minute walk.
3. Climb a flight of stairs.

Immediately after each exercise check your pulse rate again. It is important not to let too much time elapse, since the heart beat returns to normal very rapidly once the activity ceases. Write the figure down to use as a comparison against tomorrow's activities.

Unless you're in terrible shape your pulse rate will not be affected significantly by these exercises. That's why they're not effective for building cardiac endurance.

To really whip the heart into shape you must exercise it enough to raise the pulse rate about 75 percent higher than it usually goes at rest. Unless you do that, your effort will be wasted. It's like trying to make your biceps stronger by lifting weights, when the weight is no heavier than a pencil.

If you really start an endurance program, after a month or two you will find that your pulse rate, when you're at rest, will be slower than it is today. This means that the heart can perform the same task of pumping blood with less effort. That's what I mean by building endurance.

Before you start such a program and drastically change your activity level, however, there's one thing you ought to do. Get a physician to give you a stress test, also called a treadmill EKG. An EKG measures the heart's electrical activity and is a good way to diagnose heart disease. A resting EKG, which is the kind most doctors do in their offices, isn't as good as a treadmill test. The resting EKG tells what your heart is like when you're not moving, but you want to know what it's going to be like when you really stress it with exercise.

Stress tests are expensive, but they are worth the extra money. If your heart is going to have problems when you're exercising vigorously, the best place to find that out is in the doctor's office, not flat on your back on a tennis court.

Today you get the Feeling Fine point for the exercises you already did—even if they didn't raise your heart rate.

FEELING FINE POINTS
(Choose one or more from each category.)

GROWING PLEASURES
- [ ] **Skipping, cutting, and substituting with habits**
- [ ] Taking time along
- [ ] Choose your own pleasures

UNSTRESSING PLEASURES
- [ ] **Trying meditation**
- [ ] Finding a stress trigger
- [ ] Choose your own pleasure

EATING PLEASURES
- [ ] **Paying attention to your food**
- [ ] Taking control of eating cues
- [ ] Choose your own pleasure

BODY PLEASURES
- [ ] **Finding out about endurance**
- [ ] Stretching for flexibility
- [ ] Choose your own pleasure

DAY 18

Growing Pleasures

VALUE YOUR FEELINGS

"Deux cent francs," the artist said. "Forty-five dollars."

My heart pounded as I looked at the painting. It was no Van Gogh, but there on an easel in Montmartre was a painting that captured all of my feelings about Paris. Still, my practical side told me that forty-five dollars was too much money for the painting.

"Je n'ai pas l'argent," I replied, hoping the price would come down. "Thirty-five dollars," I whispered.

"Deux cent francs." And his expression said not a penny less.

I really wanted that painting. Ten dollars stood between me and a portrait of the city I loved. My feelings said "Buy!" My practical side said "Walk." I hesitated. Then I walked away.

My heart sank when he didn't call me to stop. My stomach told me the decision was all wrong. My feelings told me I had made a mistake. But I kept walking.

Five years later I returned to the exact spot. The artist was gone. The painting was gone. My feelings had been right.

Many times since then I've tried to figure out why I denied myself that painting. For months after I returned from that first trip I relived the decision, wishing I could take it back. I never got my painting, but the experience gave me a valuable lesson—I learned to pay more attention to my feelings.

It's a hard lesson to learn. All our lives we are taught to base our decisions solely on the facts, not on our feelings. We are supposed to have good reasons for everything we do. To be able to explain and justify our behavior. Feelings are supposed to be an unreliable way to measure the rightness or wrongness of what we do. Not so.

When you make some decision and then have uneasy feelings about it, it's your body's way of telling you that part of your mind is unhappy with the choice you've made.

When you win an argument with your spouse and then can't sleep all night, your feelings are trying to tell you there's something wrong with your victory.

When you buy some new clothes because someone else likes the way you look in them—but you don't —and you leave the store unhappy, your feelings are trying to tell you that you may have made a mistake.

Don't just go on feeling bad. Listen to those feelings and take them into account. You may have to change your decision, apologize, or even take something back to the store, but you'll find that you'll be feeling fine when you do.

From now on—after you've done or decided something and somehow it just doesn't feel right—you can earn a Feeling Fine point by asking yourself whether you really want to stick to that decision. It doesn't matter whether or not you end up changing your mind; the idea is to end up paying attention to your feelings.

• When you punish the kids for making too much noise and then you don't feel good, ask yourself if your body is trying to tell you you've been unfair.

• When you've been forced into making a dinner date and you immediately feel awful about it, ask yourself if unmaking the date would be the right way to feel fine again.

• When you've had some harsh words with someone and come away feeling lousy, ask yourself if saying
some kind words would make you feel better.

Give your feelings a hearing. Make them part of
your decision-making process, and chances are you'll end
up Feeling Fine.

Unstressing Pleasures

THE MEDITATION RESPONSE

If the meditation exercise you did yesterday
worked the first time you tried it, you're a better medi-
tator than I am. One week after finishing my TM course
I still had not reached "nirvana." I wanted my $125 back.
They don't return your money in TM, so I kept trying—I
practiced another week, and it finally worked. It was
worth waiting for.

What happened was something more than the
physiological changes that Dr. Benson called "the relaxation response." Those words only tell about a part of
what's going on. Meditating is a lot more than simple relaxation. That's why I prefer to call it "the meditation response."

You'll know when it happens to you. The size
and shape of your world will change. Your mind will
present you with new feelings and new sensations (some
people say it's like smoking marijuana). Your body becomes extremely cooperative. Your mind reverberates
with emptiness. Descriptions vary widely: "a natural
high," "a resonant void," "floating in the clouds," "per-
fection," "peace."

And it doesn't end there. After you finish your meditating you'll greet the world with a different face. When someone dents your car in the parking lot you'll ask how the driver feels instead of worrying about how your car looks. Sound farfetched? People said I was a changed person after I started meditating. No anger. No snapping. No tension.

Will it solve all your problems? No. Cure all your ills? No. Bring you added peace and pleasure? It should. Try it.

In fact, try it again today for ten minutes, following the instructions given yesterday, and you've earned another point for Feeling Fine.

Eating Pleasures

SERVING "RESTAURANT STYLE" AT HOME

Restaurant owners have succeeded in making eating fun because they know how to enhance the whole eating experience. They do this by wooing the eye before they please the palate. They know that food attractively served satisfies more than food eaten in pale surroundings.

Good restaurateurs do this in many ways. They choose wall and room decor with care and grace the tables with lovely linen, sparkling stemware, and fine silver. They gratify the senses even before the food is on the table. Then, when dinner does arrive, they delight you again because plates are garnished with sprigs of parsley and the food is carefully chosen for color, texture, and flavor.

Take a lesson from the experts. Learn how to make food attractive and make a little seem like a lot. Serve "restaurant style" in your own home. Here's how.

THE TABLE

1. Use a colorful tablecloth or attractive place mats.

2. Put out cloth napkins to match. If you'd rather use paper ones, buy some that are vividly colored or patterned.

3. Lay out your best silverware. Why reserve it just for company?

4. Use flowers or greenery for a centerpiece.

5. Put candles on the table. Candles don't seem ridiculous when you're paying ten to twenty dollars at a restaurant, so why feel silly about using them at home?

THE FOOD

1. Choose foods with an eye to color. Mashed potatoes, coleslaw, and filet of sole might be nutritionally balanced but they don't have much color appeal. Change the potatoes to a broiled tomato, sprinkle paprika on the fish, add some sliced green pepper and grated carrots to the coleslaw. And don't forget to be generous with the parsley. It costs little but has such a visual punch that caterers sprinkle it on everything.

2. Choose foods with different textures—soft foods contrasted with chewy or crunchy foods, raw with cooked.

THE SERVICE

1. Serve food in attractive dishes. People who cook and eat alone are often tempted to eat out of cooking pots and pans. Don't do it.

2. Don't prepare enough food for seconds. Restaurants give you just one serving and you're usually satisfied.

3. Keep serving platters out of sight in the kitchen. The desire for seconds may vanish if the food isn't in sight.

4. Serve meals in a leisurely way, one course at a time. This extends the dining hour and gives you a chance to concentrate on each dish. There is another reason for serving one course at a time, a physiological one. Once the stomach is full it sends a signal to the brain telling it "You have had enough." But that stomach signal takes twenty minutes to get to the brain. If you eat in only ten minutes, the stomach doesn't have time to tell the brain it's full. You'll eat unnecessary food, taking in more than your body needs.

One Feeling Fine point for each time you open a restaurant in your dining room.

Body Pleasures

ENDURANCE: NON-JOG YOUR WAY TO HEALTH

Although absence makes the heart grow fonder, only the right kind of exercise makes the heart grow stronger.

As we found out yesterday some exercises may be beneficial in keeping joints flexible and muscles elastic, but they're not strenuous enough to increase the heart rate and build endurance. That's why you really need to start doing some endurance exercises.

Before you begin these exercises, however, you need to find out *how much* to increase your heart rate. It's important not to increase it too much. Scientists have learned that there is a different safe maximum heart rate for each of us, based on our sex and age. You can find out your safe maximum heart rate by asking your doctor or the Fitness Director at the local YMCA. (You might also talk to the director about the fitness program they have. No one does it as well as the "Y.")

No doubt the first endurance exercise that comes to mind is jogging. Jogging is certainly one of the best, but there are many other enjoyable ways you can elevate your heart rate and strengthen your cardiovascular system. Take a look at these.

Rock-and-Roll Dancing. You don't need good weather or special equipment; all you need is soul. Buy some records or tune in a rock station. If you haven't tried it, I guarantee you'll find lively and sustained dancing to rock music can really increase the heart rate. Be sure to begin slowly, dancing three or four minutes at a time, then gradually build up until you can dance fifteen to twenty minutes without stopping.

Swimming. This is an excellent endurance-building exercise. It is especially beneficial for people with joint problems such as arthritis.

Bike Riding. Pedaling fast for ten or fifteen blocks will bring anyone's heart rate up. If you ride on a level area, pedal in high gear and pedal faster.

Stationary Bike Riding. If dogs, traffic, and carbon monoxide bother you and you can't find bike paths or quiet residential streets to ride on, try a stationary bike. Good stationary bikes feature devices with adjustable pedal resistance. The greater the resistance, the harder you pedal and the faster your heart will go. An indoor bike can be used year 'round—and you can put it outside when the weather is good. If you place yours near the television or stereo, you can entertain yourself while turning wheels. (Since exercise cycles are rather expensive, try renting before you buy.)

Skipping Rope. This is not just child's play. Ask any boxer. It's ideal not only for building cardiac endurance but it's also great for legs, arms, shoulders, and the upper body. It's easy to learn, equipment is cheap, and you can take it with you wherever you go (although the other guests may complain if you use it in your hotel room). To add variety you can skip to music or jump rope with a friend. Once you get the hang of it, ten minutes of skipping will give you as much exercise as thirty minutes of jogging. Be sure the rope is long enough to reach up under your armpits when you stand on it. Also, a soft surface (carpet or lawn) is better than hard; if you do jump on a hard surface, wear shoes with cushioned soles. Just jump high enough for the rope to go under your feet (about an inch off the floor is enough). Flex your ankles, knees, and hips slightly. Land on the balls of your feet for a light landing. Begin by jumping one or two minutes several times a day. Add a minute each week until you can do ten to fifteen minutes.

Basketball, Handball, Squash. These games are good endurance builders but require other players. Be sure to keep the game going long enough and play hard enough to keep your heart beating at an increased rate for several minutes at a time.

Before you begin any of these endurance-building exercises you should be aware of these precautions.

1. Warm up gradually by limbering, stretching, or walking. Don't fling yourself into the exercise with a burst of energy. When you are sedentary your muscles are supplied with about 12 percent of your blood. During vigorous activity they require 88 percent. The older you

are, the more time it takes to adjust to that change. So if you are not in very good condition be sure to warm up slowly.

2. End gradually, too. Don't totally collapse into an armchair when you're through. All athletes, fighters, and even race horses walk or hop around after fully exerting themselves. This keeps the blood from pooling in the legs and prevents fainting. Stretch again before you sit down.

3. Wait for at least an hour after eating before exercising vigorously so that you don't disturb the digestive process.

4. Exercise for a reasonable length of time. Don't play to exhaustion. If you can't talk while you're exercising, you're exercising too hard for your heart. As your endurance increases, you'll gradually increase the time you can exercise without exhaustion.

5. If you experience pain, nausea, or dizziness, stop.

6. Exercise regularly. Try to schedule yourself for at least three times a week. Otherwise you'll lose the endurance you've built up.

7. To repeat, be sure to check with your physician before beginning any endurance program to be sure you can tolerate it safely. Get a stress EKG test.

For other exercise ideas write your local chapter of the American Heart Association or to the President's Council on Physical Fitness and Sports (400 Sixth St., S.W., Washington, D.C. 20201) for their suggestions.

For using any of these techniques to get started on a heart-building program give yourself a Feeling Fine point.

FEELING FINE POINTS
(Choose one or more from each category.)

GROWING PLEASURES
☐ **Paying attention to your feelings**
☐ Solving problems through guided imagery
☐ Choose two of your own pleasures
UNSTRESSING PLEASURES
☐ **Trying meditation**
☐ Relieving pain through guided imagery
☐ Try two of your own pleasures
EATING PLEASURES
☐ **Opening a "restaurant" in your dining room**
☐ Getting fiber in your food
☐ Pick two of your own pleasures
BODY PLEASURES
☐ **Helping your heart grow stronger**
☐ Moving the Feldenkrais way
☐ Select two of your own pleasures

DAY 19

Growing Pleasures

SURROUNDING YOURSELF WITH PLEASURE

Check any freeway out of Los Angeles (or any big city) on a Friday evening and you'll always find the same thing—the road is jammed with people trying to get to more pleasant surroundings. They're headed for the mountains, the desert, the beach—anywhere but the place they're in.

We've all got special places we'd like to be, but most of us can't go there as often as we'd like. That doesn't mean we have to do without the pleasures of our special places.

If you can't go to the mountains, why not bring the mountains to you? I can't go skiing as often as I'd like so I bring the ski resorts home. I've covered the walls of the garage with ski posters. Every time I go to the car I'm surrounded with the pleasures of skiing, even though I can't be there.

My publisher loves the Colorado River, so he covered the walls of his office and his bedroom with pictures of his raft trip on the river. Now he can't look up from a manuscript or go to bed without reliving some of the pleasures of that place.

One doctor I know loves to fish. You won't find any medical plaques in his office. The walls are covered with pictures of fish. Another friend loves to visit historic places. His office looks like an antique shop.

You can turn your everyday environment into a place of pleasure, too. You don't have to hire an expensive decorator—just turn your memory on and let your imagination go to work.

Is camping your thing? Put a Coleman lantern and a canteen in your office—remind yourself of campfire fun everytime you go to work.

Tennis your pleasure? Make a mobile or a sculpture out of some tired tennis balls or hang a racquet on your wall—score a point for pleasure everytime you enter the room.

Is the desert your source of joy? Plant a cactus garden outside your living room window.

Blow up a photo of your favorite trip and place it where you can see it every day. Move the pictures of people you like out of your wallet and onto your walls so you can take pleasure from their company all the time.

Get involved with your environment. Surround yourself with things that please you and you'll feel more pleasant. Remind yourself of things that relax you and you'll feel less tense. It's visual imagery all over again, but a little less is left to the imagination.

Make a list of the things that make you feel good and then find a way to make them part of your surroundings.

Move some pleasures from the corners of your memory to the center of your attention and give yourself another point for Feeling Fine.

Unstressing Pleasures

THE MEDITATION RESPONSE: DOUBLING THE TIME

If one pill is good, two must be better. Wrong. But unlike medicine, meditation gets better when you double the dose. Doubling the meditation time doubles the benefits. For reasons no one really understands, meditation is much more effective when practiced on two different occasions during the day.

Your challenge for today? Double up. If you've been practicing the meditation response once a day, double the dose. Once in the morning, once in the late afternoon or early evening. Stretch your ten minutes into fifteen or twenty and expand the benefits even more.

I know what most of you are saying right now: "Twenty minutes, twice a day? I don't have the time."

Believe it or not, most of us *do* have that much extra time in the day which can be used for meditation. It may be well disguised, but it's there. Here are some tips on times you can find to squeeze in the extra "dose."

Scheduled Breaks. You may have several every day—coffee breaks, lunch hour, minutes between meetings, even "john" breaks. Return from your lunch hour early. Use the time for the meditation response. If you work at home, drop one chore from your morning schedule and meditate. Let the breakfast dishes wait and do them with the lunch or dinner dishes. Don't dust. Don't vacuum. Probably no one will know the difference. But *you* will feel it.

Leisure Time. Cut your television viewing time short by 600 seconds. Devote less time to reading the paper. Bowl three games instead of four.

Substitution Time. Instead of spending half an hour on the phone listening to your friends' complaints, use the phone only for pleasantries and spend the rest of your "phone time" meditating. If you're often faced with a pack of woes when you come home, park your car a block away and meditate before you get home. When you finally do open the door, you'll find yourself much better able to cope with what you find there.

Waiting Time. Everybody has it. You can practice meditating while waiting to get on the golf course or tennis court. One of the best ways to find meditating time is to be early for an appointment. Doctor not ready? Meditate. Friend hasn't shown up yet? Meditate.

Sleeping Time. If nothing else works, get up ten minutes earlier in the morning.

The ideal meditation time is twenty minutes, twice a day. If you feel you're being asked for the impossible with ten, you may wonder how you're ever going to manage twenty. It's a problem for everyone, but it's a problem worth solving. Perhaps you could try it for the first time on a weekend, when there are more leisure hours. Meditate twenty minutes in the morning and another twenty in the evening on both Saturday and Sunday. See what happens. Then incorporate as many of these twenty-minute slots as you can into the rest of your week.

In time, meditation may become a part of your life. You may become so conditioned that you'll be able to meditate not only in a quiet, darkened room but in a cab rushing to an appointment, in a corner of an airline terminal, even in Grand Central Station.

Try meditating again today. Twice! And give yourself two Feeling Fine points for doubling the meditation response.

Eating
Pleasures

EATING OUT AND
FEELING FINE

As we said yesterday, eating "restaurant style" at home is fun. But eating "restaurant style" in a restaurant is even more fun. It's a joy to let someone else prepare the food and clean up afterward. It's a pleasure to have someone else wait on you.

There are times, however, when we spoil the fun of a restaurant—by eating too much. We see the tantalizing descriptions of foods on the menu. We smell the food as it's being served to others at nearby tables. And we lose our heads. We order more than we really should.

Does that sound like a familiar problem? Here are some tips to help you avoid that trap in the future.

Order à la Carte. Choose foods you love, so that you can enjoy them to gourmet satisfaction. Stay away from the low-cost specials and seven-course dinners that come with "everything" included. It's the "everything" you need to avoid if you want to keep your health. The bargain dinners are no bargain if they end up as extra inches on your waistline. Try an appetizer as your main dish. The portion is smaller, and so is the price.

Substitute. Tomatoes for creamed corn, salad for sandwiches, clear soup for potatoes. Most good restaurants will allow substitutions. If the one you patronize won't do that, the next time you go out substitute restaurants.

Cut Portions. Ask your waiter or waitress for half portions. If you must order a full portion, ask them to put half on your plate and half in a "doggie bag" *before* they serve it to you. You'll never be tempted by the half you can't see. You'll save calories, and you'll have tomorrow's lunch in a bag.

Share the Load. If you have a partner at your meal, order one main course with two dishes—half the calories, half the price, twice the fun.

Send the Bread. Far away. Don't leave a full bread basket on the table. Take one piece and then have the basket removed. Why tempt yourself throughout the meal? Don't forget to send the butter dish away, too.

Leave Some Food. Don't eat all the food on your plate just because you're paying for it. You'll still pay whether you eat it or leave it. If you're not really hungry enough to eat it all, don't force yourself.

Having fun in a restaurant depends on *how* you eat as well as *what* you eat. Here are some "how-to" tips that can make restaurant visits more enjoyable.

Ask for a Nice Table. Don't be bashful. Tell the host or hostess that you are willing to wait if necessary. Why spend your evening in the corner listening to the dishes being washed instead of enjoying the ocean view?

Take Your Time. Make sure you have enough time to enjoy a leisurely meal. After you are seated, ask the waiter or waitress to serve slowly and to bring only one course at a time.

Complain, If Necessary. Make sure you get what you paid for. Don't be afraid to complain or send food back. If you wanted cold food, you could prepare it at home for half the price. Be polite but firm. Above all, be happy.

Next time you go out to eat, put this restaurant plan into action and you'll earn yourself another Feeling Fine point.

Body
Pleasures

ENDURANCE: JOG YOUR WAY
TO HEALTH

"It's better than drugs, better than alcohol, and —sometimes—it's better than sex."

Believe it or not, that's the way one avid runner described jogging. Personally, I can't go along with *everything* he said, but I do agree that jogging can be a lot of fun. The trouble is, most people can't get into it enough to enjoy it. Whenever I ask them why not, I get the same answers:

"It's no fun."

"It's dangerous."

"It's a waste of time."

Here's how I respond to those comments:

Jogging is fun when you do it right. It feels good and it makes you look good. That's fun. When you jog you meet interesting people and see interesting things. That's fun. You gain a sense of accomplishment and pride. That's fun. You gain new stamina and new strength. That's fun, too.

Jogging is good for your health. When you jog regularly and in a sensible program you greatly increase the ability of your heart to endure stress. That's not dangerous. You decrease the amount of work your heart has to do because you increase its efficiency with every stroke. That's not dangerous. Jogging builds leg muscles and trims waistlines. That's not dangerous. That's good for your health.

Jogging is more than just running. Ask anyone who jogs regularly and he or she will tell you that it is definitely not a waste of time. Some will talk about the way it relaxes them. Others will tell you they solve problems while they run. Down at the track where I do my running (not as regularly as I'd like) there's a guy who listens to the news when he jogs. He carries a little radio on his wrist, just like Dick Tracy.

I'm not going to try to make a jogger out of you today. You don't have to run a mile to get your point for the day. All you have to do is think about it. If it sounds interesting at all, the following tips will be helpful to you.

1. Get into a sensible jogging program. Some of the best ones in the country are run by the YMCA. Call your local "Y" for more information. If they can't help you, write the National Jogging Association (1910 K Street, N.W., Suite 202, Washington, D.C. 20006) for the names of jogging groups near you.

2. As we mentioned on Day 17, get an exercise stress test before you make *any* drastic change in the amount of physical activity you do.

3. Start your jogging program slowly, gradually building your ability to run longer and faster. Rushing the program endangers your health and spoils the fun.

4. Jog at least three times a week. If you allow more than three days to elapse between each session you'll lose some of the benefits from the last run.

5. Buy special "training" shoes. They have cushioned soles, good arch support, and specially designed heels to avoid tendon and ankle problems. Most injuries are due to poor shoes. Ordinary tennis shoes should *never* be used.

6. Jog on a soft surface. Grass is great, rubber and dirt tracks are fine. Asphalt or concrete creates too much strain on the shins and lower back unless you wear shoes especially designed for those surfaces.

7. Jog heel-to-toe. If you jog on just your toes, you'll put too much strain on your calf muscles.

8. Jog in the morning or early evening. Going out too late in the day may overstimulate you and make it hard to fall asleep at night.

9. Jog in different locations. Just as playing different golf courses adds interest to the game, varying your jogging locale will add to your pleasure.

Just for thinking about jogging, give yourself a Feeling Fine point. (This may be the easiest point to earn in the whole book.)

FEELING FINE POINTS
(Choose one or more from each category.)

GROWING PLEASURES

☐ **Putting pleasure where you can see it**

☐ Keeping control of your habits

☐ Choose two of your own pleasures

UNSTRESSING PLEASURES

☐ **Meditating a bit more**

☐ Taking control of your stress

☐ Pick two of your own pleasures

EATING PLEASURES

☐ **Dining out**

☐ Dining in as if you were dining out

☐ Choose two of your own pleasures

BODY PLEASURES

☐ **Helping your heart work better**

☐ Limbering up your limbs

☐ Try two of your own pleasures

DAY 20

Growing
Pleasures

RESPONDING TO THE MOMENT

Last year on a vacation in Vermont I was walking up the steps of the State Capitol building when it hit me—a wave of excitement from somewhere within—a good feeling. I had returned to visit my boyhood home, and I was surging with pleasure. I couldn't contain myself. Standing next to an old cannon, with one hand on the barrel, I began a speech.

"Fellow Vermonters," I shouted to the strangers walking by, "your long-lost son has returned. I have come home."

Making that speech in my shorts and tennis shoes I know I looked and sounded rather silly, but I wasn't feeling silly. I was feeling fine. Very fine.

As I continued my speech I couldn't help but notice the wide variety of reactions from my audience. The natives stared in disbelief. Douglas clapped, Steven laughed, Valerie blushed, and Priscilla snapped pictures.

What was behind my bizarre behavior? Had I gone crazy? No, I had gone truly sane. I was feeling real emotion, genuine excitement. And I was permitting those feelings to reach the surface and come out in action. I was responding to the moment, and I was feeling fine.

Life has many special moments, times when your feelings are trying to get in touch with you. Don't shut them off. Let them through—even if they are asking you to change your plans on less than a moment's notice, skip down the street instead of walking, or hug a friend you've never hugged before. The more you let your feelings through, the more such moments you'll enjoy.

You don't have to learn any tricks to do it. Just think back to childhood. When the music played, we danced—no matter who was watching. When the heroine died in the Saturday matinée, we cried—no matter who was watching. When the band played, we sang—no matter who was listening. Why did we ever stop such spontaneity? Probably because when we were children, grownups said it was taboo. We were too noisy, too embarrassing; it wasn't manly, or feminine, or something or other.

It's time to regain that lovely quality of childhood—the ability to respond to any moment. It's never too late to experience your feelings.

Next time you're stuck in traffic and the radio plays your favorite song, sing—no matter how many motorists may notice.

Next time you feel like shouting during a ball game, shout—even if you're the only one rooting for the visiting team.

Next time you feel like kissing your spouse, do it—especially if the kids are in the room. You'll show them how great it feels to be spontaneous.

> Shout your happiness.
> Shed your tears.
> Break a taboo.
> Dance without inhibition.
> Reach out with affection.
> Listen to your feelings.
> Respond to the moment.

Whatever you're feeling, let it through and you'll always be able to give yourself another point for Feeling Fine.

Unstressing Pleasures

DERAILING STRESS

When something upsets you at noon, doing guided imagery at five that evening is better than doing nothing at all. But it's not as good as doing guided imagery at 12:01.

When something upsets you at bedtime, meditation the next morning is better than no meditation at all. But it's not as good as meditation at midnight. The key is: the sooner the better.

For three weeks you've been learning and using techniques which help your body to cancel the effects of stress *after* it occurs. If you're like most readers, you've used the techniques whenever it was convenient, not necessarily when you needed them the most. When do you need them the most? Right at the time the stress is occurring. That's why—starting today—you're going to stop stress in its tracks. You're going to cancel it out as soon as it occurs. Whenever you can you'll cancel it *before* it starts. And each time you do, give yourself another Feeling Fine point.

It doesn't matter which technique you use. Expect trouble with the boss? Close your eyes and picture yourself in Hawaii and see how cool you are when the trouble (or the boss) arrives. Missed the bus? Sit down on the bench and enjoy some autogenics. Burned the roast? Meditate your stress away before dinner.

You may have to make your stress-reducing activity briefer than usual, but that's okay. If you do it at the time stress is occurring, it doesn't take as much to cancel the effects of stress on your body. If you do it before the stress arrives, your body will never even feel the stress.

Today and for the rest of your life, stop stress before it happens, deal with it when it occurs, cancel it after it has taken place—and congratulate yourself for taking an active role in Feeling Fine.

Eating Pleasures

CREATIVE EATING

Are you in a food rut?

Is it eggs for breakfast, a sandwich for lunch, fish on Friday, and roast on Sunday?

When you have wine, is it always red wine with meat and white wine with fish?

When you go out, is it soup and salad, steak and potatoes, apple pie and ice cream?

What a bore! You are missing out on one of the great experiences life has to offer. It's called "creative eating," and you don't have to break any Feeling Fine rules to do it. The pleasures of creative eating will be obvious as soon as you hear about it, so here's how you do it.

Try New Routines. Chicken for breakfast and eggs for dinner. Dessert before the main course. White wine with meat. A sandwich for supper and lasagna for lunch. Take a lesson from the twenty-four-hour coffee shops. Be willing to eat anything at any time and everything you eat will taste new and more interesting, just by changing the time of day.

Try New Foods. Okra, guava, mangoes, plantains, bok choy, mustard greens, artichokes, jicama, fennel, rutabaga, rabbit, squid, codfish. Are these foods just words in a dictionary or flavors in your memory? Why not get familiar with some foods you haven't tried? Try each one once. If you don't like it, don't have it again.

Try New Recipes. Expand your repertoire. Surprise your family and friends. You don't have to experiment with an entire meal—try one new dish at a time. You may pleasantly surprise yourself.

Add Something New to the Old. Bean sprouts to salads, seeds to soups, mushrooms to meats, chicken to pizza. Make up your own as you go. Don't forget that someone had to experiment with melon wrapped in ham before the world made it a delicacy.

Try New Restaurants. Even if you love Italian food, you don't have to go to the same restaurant all the time. Try a new one, or return to a neglected favorite. Don't be afraid to cross some international borders. Experiment with ethnic restaurants. Don't be surprised if you run into some pretty strange flavors, so ask for small samples. Sometimes they've got a little extra in the kitchen. Look for things to enjoy, not to criticize. A whole world of tastes awaits you.

Do some creative eating today, eat healthier every day, and earn a Feeling Fine point every time you sit down at the table.

Body Pleasures

DANCING: YOU GOT RHYTHM

When I started on local television in Los Angeles in 1975, we needed a picture to symbolize the "Feeling Fine program. We wanted something without words that would instantaneously communicate the idea of feeling fine. One of the top graphic designers in town was commissioned to do the job. Before he went to the drawing board he spent several days learning about the program and about me. A week later he returned with a picture that has remained my logo ever since.

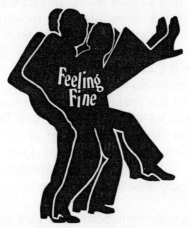

Why is a dancing couple the symbol of "Feeling Fine"? Because it represents so many of the individual elements of the "Feeling Fine" program all joined together. The spontaneity of "Responding to the Moment." The freedom of "Longer and Looser." The warmth of "Reaching out with Affection."

That's why I've chosen to end the Body Pleasures section of this book with dancing. That's why—to earn your point today—you'll dance. Don't worry if you "don't know how to dance." Everyone knows how. People were dancing for thousands of years before Arthur Murray came along. They never needed lessons, and you won't either—because dancing is a natural response to the sounds around us and the rhythm within us.

If you want proof, just watch children. They'll dance at the drop of a hat or the sound of a drum. Why

don't grownups do the same? I don't know for sure, but
my guess is that whenever they did, some square came
along and told them to stop acting like children.

Don't worry about today's dance just because
you don't have a partner. You don't need one to dance.
Take a look at one of the TV programs where all the kids
are dancing to rock or soul music and watch them closely.
They're so wrapped up in their own movements that it's
hard to tell which partner belongs to whom. One other
thing you'll notice: they're all having a fantastic time.
They're all Feeling Fine.

You can be Feeling Fine, too, in as little time as it
takes to turn on the radio or put on a record. When the
music comes on, let the dance come out. Don't be bashful—respond to the moment! Clap your hands, dance
for joy. Is there anyone around? Don't be embar-
rassed—reach out with affection! Never did it before?
Don't let that stop you—set new limits!

Say it with your body, and give yourself a fun-
filled Feeling Fine point.

FEELING FINE POINTS

GROWING PLEASURES

☐ **You're on your own**

UNSTRESSING PLEASURES

☐ **You're on your own**

EATING PLEASURES

☐ **You're on your own**

BODY PLEASURES

☐ **You're on your own**

A Note
from the Author

My program is over. Yours is just beginning. Twenty days of Feeling Fine lie behind you. A lifetime of Feeling Fine lies ahead. You don't need my program to continue—develop your own.

Make pleasure your constant companion. Pleasure your body by caring for it. Pleasure yourself by caring. Whenever you can, wherever you are—be good to yourself.

You'll feel fine forever.

Art Ulene

Feeling Fine Reading

GROWING PLEASURES

Fast, Julius. *The Pleasure Book*. New York: Stein and Day, 1975.

Fensterheim, Herbert, and Jean Baer. *Don't Say Yes When You Want to Say No*. New York: David McKay, 1975.

Garfield, Patricia. *Creative Dreaming*. New York: Simon and Schuster, 1975.

Huxley, Laura Archera. *You Are Not the Target*. New York: Avon, 1963.

Missiledine, Hugh. *Your Inner Child of the Past*. New York: Simon and Schuster, 1963.

Robbins, Jhan, and Dave Fisher. *How to Make and Break Habits*. New York: Dell, 1973.

Samuels, Mike, and Hal Bennett. *The Well Body Book*. New York: Random House, 1973.

Viscott, David. *The Language of Feeling*. New York: Arbor House, 1976.

UNSTRESSING PLEASURES

Akins, W. R., and George Nurnberg. *How to Meditate without Attending a TM Class*. New York: Amjon, 1976.

Benson, Herbert. *The Relaxation Response*. New York: William Morrow, 1975.

Jacobson, Edmund. *You Must Relax*. New York: McGraw-Hill, 1962.

Lindemann, Hannes. *Relieve Tension the Autogenic Way.* New York: Peter H. Wyden, 1973.

Pellettier, Kenneth. *Mind as Healer, Mind as Slayer.* New York: Delacorte, 1977.

Samuels, Mike, and Nancy Samuels. *Seeing with the Mind's Eye.* New York: Random House, 1975.

Selye, Hans. *Stress without Distress.* New York: Lippincott, 1974.

Shealy, Norman. *90 Days to Self-Health.* New York: Dial, 1977.

———. © Biogenic tapes available from The Pain and Health Rehabilitation Center, Route 2, La Crosse, Wis. 54601.

EATING PLEASURES

Amit, Zalman, and E. Ann Sutherland. *Stay Slim for Good.* New York: Walker, 1976.

Ashley, Richard, and Heidi Duggal. *Dictionary of Nutrition.* New York: St. Martin's Press, 1976.

Jordan, Henry A.; Leonard S. Levitz; and Gordon M. Kimbrell. *Eating Is Okay!* New York: Rawson, 1976.

Kraus, Barbara. *1975 Calorie Guide to Brand Names and Basic Foods.* New York: New American Library, 1975.

Mahoney, Michael J., and Kathryn Mahoney. *Permanent Weight Control.* New York: Norton, 1976.

Reuben, David. *Save-Your-Life Diet: High Fiber Protection from Six of the Most Serious Diseases of Civilization.* New York: Random House, 1975.

Sabry, Zak, and Ruth Fremes. *Nutriscore: The Rate-Yourself Plan for Better Nutrition*. New York: Two Continents, 1976.

U.S. Department of Agriculture. Bulletin #8, "Composition of Foods." Washington, D.C.: U.S. Government Printing Office, 1975.

BODY PLEASURES

Anderson, Bob. *Stretching*. Englewood, Colo., 1975.

Boston Women's Health Book Collective. *Our Bodies, Ourselves*. New York: Simon and Schuster, 1976.

Cooper, Kenneth H. *Aerobics*. New York: M. Evans, 1968.

Cooper, Mildred, and Kenneth H. Cooper. *Aerobics for Women*. New York: M. Evans, 1972.

Diagram Group. *Man's Body: An Owner's Manual*. New York: Two Continents, 1976.

Downing, George. *The Massage Book*. New York: Random House, 1972.

Feldenkrais, Moshe. *Awareness through Movement*. New York: Harper and Row, 1972.

Friedmann, Lawrence W., and Lawrence Galton. *Freedom from Backaches*. New York: Simon and Schuster, 1973.

Gullers, K. W., and Berit Brattnas. *Fit for Fun: A Swedish Massage*. New York: Van Nostrand Reinhold, 1974.

Inkeles, Gordon, and Murray Todris. *The Art of Sensual Massage*. San Francisco: Straight Arrow, 1972.

Jampol, Hyman. *The Weekend Athlete's Way to a Pain-Free Monday*. Los Angeles: J. P. Tarcher, 1973.

Kostrubala, Thaddeus. *The Joy of Running.* New York: Lippincott, 1976.

Morehouse, Laurence E., and Leonard Gross. *Total Fitness in 30 Minutes a Week.* New York: Simon and Schuster, 1975.

Royal Canadian Air Force Exercise Plans for Physical Fitness. New York: Simon and Schuster, 1962.

Sassoon, Beverly, and Vidal Sassoon. *A Year of Beauty and Health.* New York: Simon and Schuster, 1975.

Skolnik, Peter L. *Jump Rope!* New York: Workman, 1974.

Smith, Ann. *Stretch.* New York: Cornerstone Library, 1969.

Unger, Len. *Walking: The Perfect Exercise.* San Luis Obispo, Calif.: Impact, 1976.

Vickery, Donald M., and James F. Fries. *Take Care of Yourself.* Reading, Mass: Addison-Wesley, 1976.